Welcome to your healing!

It is time to put on your armor of God. He is our protection. When pain hits us like our souls have been knocked out of our bodies; He Grabs us, Heals us, Restores us, Secures us, Regenerates us, all out of the pure love He has for us.

Buckle your seat belt and get ready for the ride! This journey may be bumpy, but have patience with yourself and don't give up. You deserve this healing!

Maryam Khalilah xoxo

MEET YOUR COACH

Maryam K. Muhammad is the creator and founder of the Heal Thy Life Center, a non-profit foundation dedicated to educating women and children on living healthier lifestyles. As a gifted orator, motivational speaker, and published author, Mrs. Muhammad has addressed audiences of all sizes; from small, intimate circles to audiences of nearly a thousand. Her inspiring words offer practical guidance for women and girls in a variety of contexts and have been known to empower the listener to make changes for the better.

One of Maryam's many passions is empowering women professionally. She has organized and hosted several networking events for entrepreneurs, served on various entrepreneur panels, provided coaching for first time business owners, and more. She has accomplished all of these things while hosting her own radio show and expanding Heal Thy Life in both the community and with businesses.

Her work has placed her in high demand and taken her all across the country to share her skill set and passion. More importantly, her travels have afforded her multiple opportunities to partner with other organizations, schools, and private circles to touch the lives of women and young people in a variety of urban communities.

The release of her highly anticipated book The Power to Break Generational Pain (2020) is a response to multiple requests to capture her words. The book is a collection of reflections, healing, affirmations, and "AHA!" moments that the author has experienced while working with women. It is an additional and invaluable tool that Mrs. Muhammad uses to continue her divine mission as a catalyst for the empowerment of women.

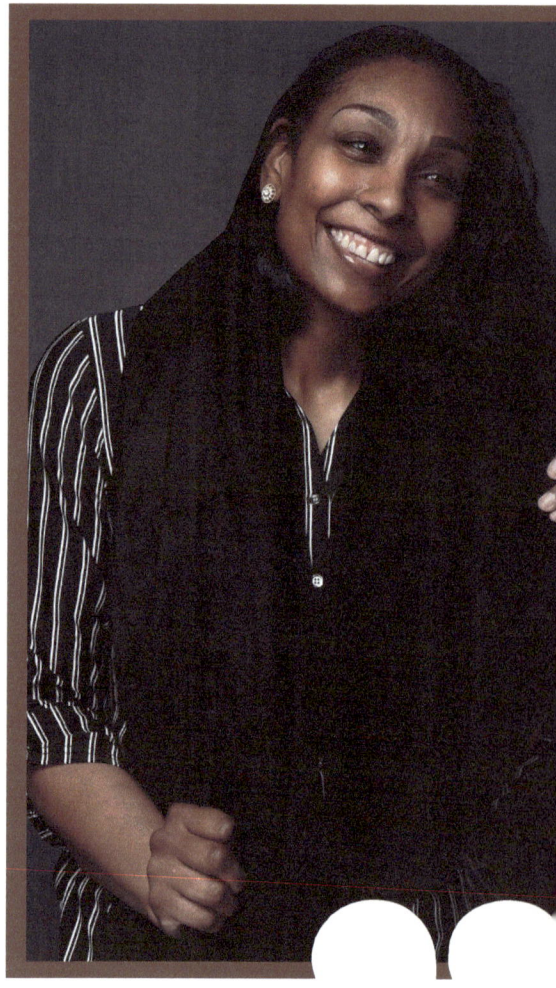

You can dream and you can vision. If it stays in your mind, it will never become a reality.

Maryam Khalilah xoxo

MY PROMISE
TO YOU

The healing process isn't always
easy. In this workbook I will give
you tools to assist you with your
healing process. The goal is to
help you stay on task until you
reach the desired destination.

The promise from my heart is to
give to you, what God has given
to me. Let's start your process!

BEGINNING ASSESSMENT

Take this brief assessment to see where you are before you begin this workbook.

	YES	NO
Do you ever feel you've been affected by fear, anxiety or panic?	YES	NO
Have you ever felt emotional pain that was inflicted on you by others or yourself?	YES	NO
Have you ever felt overwhelmed by your surrounding circumstances?	YES	NO
Do you experience restless nights?	YES	NO
Have you ever experienced doubt and depression?	YES	NO
Do you believe you can be healed?	YES	NO

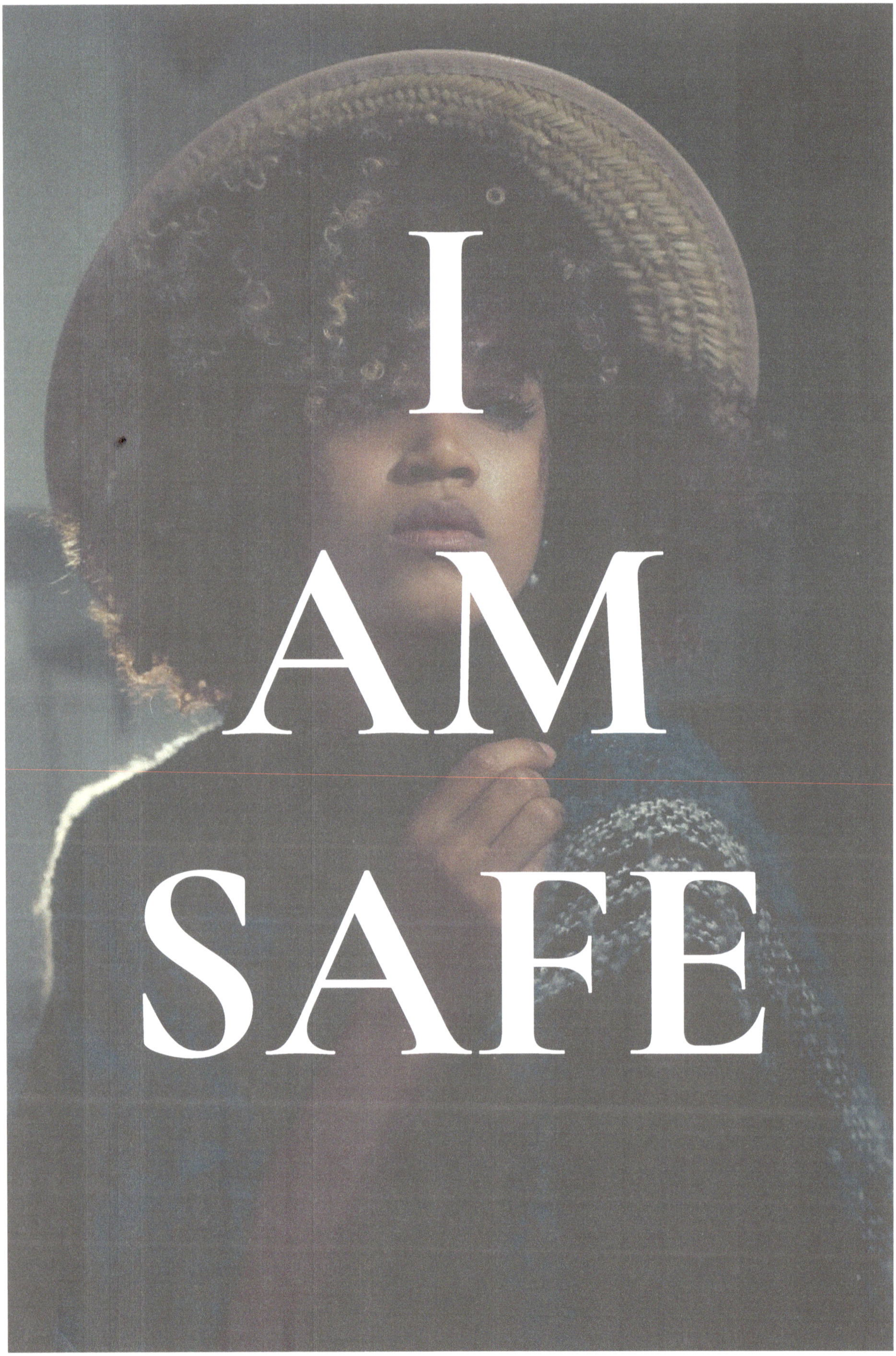

CREATING A HEALTHY MINDSET!

You have to constantly feed yourself positive thoughts, especially if you are in an environment where negativity dwells. If someone is constantly feeding you doubt, words that fuel your insecurities, words that create depression and scars of pain, you have to work double time to deflect that negative energy. You have to prepare your mind for the battlefield you walk through everyday. Establish your heaven in the midst of Satan's hell.

Experts say that it takes 21 days to break a bad habit. It also takes 21 days to make a new habit. Our biggest challenge as women is our thinking. My desire is for you to build the new habit of seeing and affirming yourself in value - EVERY DAY!
In the 21-day Affirmation Assignment, you will open your mind to receive a new way of thinking. Take the courageous step to retrain your thoughts. As a result, completing the rest of this book will become easier. Believe that!

THREE-STEP PROCESS

Before beginning any module, you must complete the Three-Step Process. This process is to help you enter into the state of being for healing.

STEP ONE...

Settle into a comfortable place and breathe mindfully. Rest for two to three minutes. You should begin to feel relaxed.

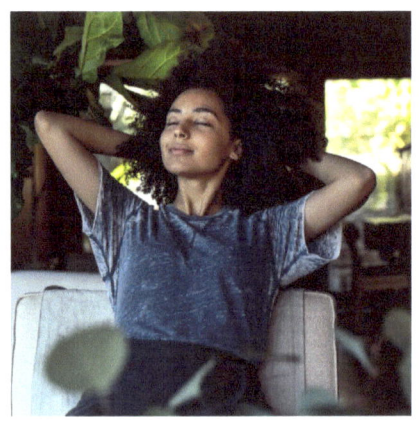

STEP TWO...

Pick an area of your body to focus on for another two to three minutes. (forehead, toes, lips, hands, etc.) Keep controlling your breathing.

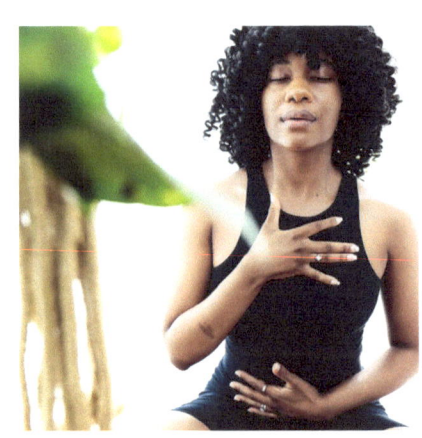

STEP THREE...

Say to yourself,
I am ready to heal.
I am ready to grow.
I am ready to become my best self!

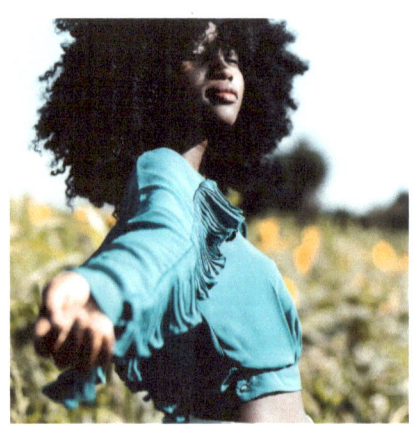

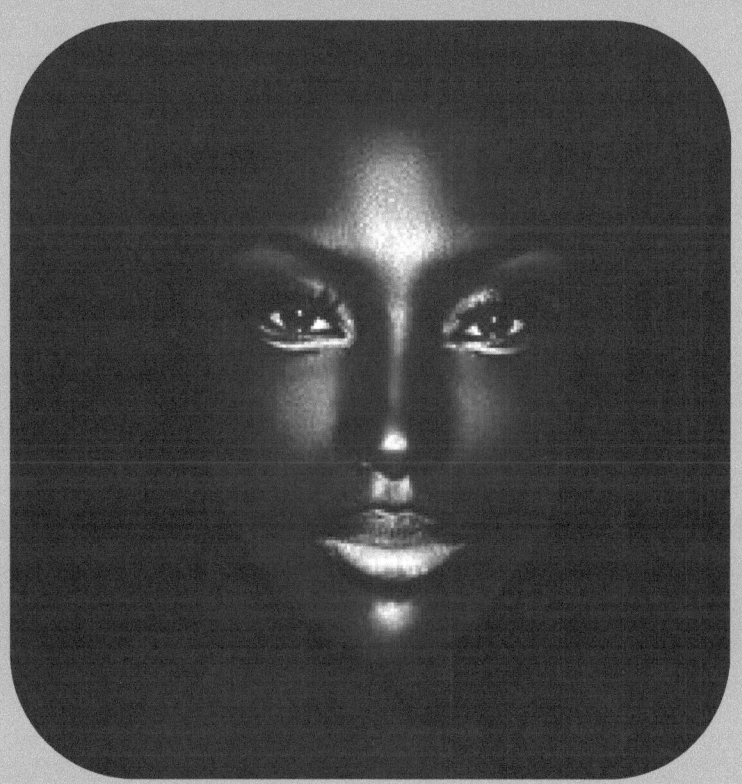

In the beginning, out of triple darkness God created Himself & next in creation was me! I am shaped and fashioned by His mind. When He breathed life into me, the essence of His spirit entered into my flesh. He looked into my eyes and fed me His word, He wrapped His arms around me embracing His companion. I layed my head on His chest at night experiencing protection, comfort and security. I inspired His creation of the sun, the planets and creatures of the earth. I stood with Him side by side. I complimented His mind. I AM THE WOMB ALL MEN COME THROUGH, I AM GOD'S CO-CREATOR, I AM THE SECOND SELF OF GOD!

MATURING YOUR THINKING INTO A HIGHER LEVEL

Develop your thinking by feeding yourself positive thoughts, words of strength and encouragement. Always remember, doubt creates resistance that feeds fear. This ultimately communicates to you that it's easier to make an excuse in the place of a sensible response.

Practice taking responsibility for your actions or creating new things. Living a purpose-filled life calls for developing an adventurous spirit. You will encounter difficulties, pain, success and much more. The more you become familiar with how powerful your mind is, the more you will begin to live on purpose.

I HAVE THE POWER TO COMPLETE THIS STEP BECAUSE.......

_____

_____

_____

_____

_____

Stimulate your mind and soul with the words of God. Stay focused on Him who has given you your purpose and watch your energy maximize.

AFFIRMING THE NEW YOU

CREATE FOUR DIFFERENT SETS OF AFFIRMATIONS.

I am open to receive.
I am ready to change for the better.
I believe in myself.
I deserve this.
I am committed to self-growth.
I am confident I can do this.
I am taking control of my life today.

I am worth all of the blessings I will receive.
I am strong enough to fight through my trials.
I am endurance.
I am equipped to handle the pain that accompanies growth.
I am worthy because God breathed the breath of life in

GOD

LOVE

STRENGTH

ENCOURAGEMENT

ANALYZING SELF

WHAT DO YOU THINK OF YOURSELF?

_____

_____

In this section you will list the positive and negative things you think about yourself. Be honest with yourself. Keep in mind, the goal of this exercise is not to beat up on yourself, but instead to acknowledge your good and pull out and identify what you need to fix.

NEGATIVES   POSITIVES

GETTING TO THE ROOT

Write down your negative thoughts. Then, list who fed these thoughts to you. Did you feed these thoughts to yourself or did someone else tell you these things? What actions or events stimulated these thoughts? Lastly, write how fear plays a role in and with your ability to change the thoughts.

NEGATIVE THOUGHTS

WHO FED THEM TO ME

WHAT STIMULATES THEM

FEAR

COUNTER THOSE THOUGHTS

In this section you are to list your negative thoughts in the left column. In the right column, list positive thoughts that you will use to counter those negative thoughts when they come up.

NEGATIVE THOUGHTS   POSITIVE THOUGHTS

CYCLE OF THOUGHTS DIAGRAM

FEED ON GOD'S
WORD

RELAX AND
BREATHE

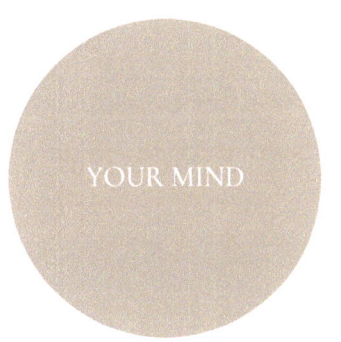

YOUR MIND

CREATE POSITIVE
THOUGHTS

CREATE POSITIVE
THOUGHTS

FEED ON
AFFIRMATIONS

Our thoughts operate on frequencies. These frequencies reflect the rate at which something occurs and they are calculated in seconds. Thought moves at the speed of 24 billion miles per second on average. Our universe communicates with us through these frequencies.

We must master the frequencies of our minds.

NOTES

ELIMINATE EXCUSES

Don't let excuses become your reality. Learn to identify the difference between an excuse and a reason. For some of us, excuses have shaped and molded our lives. They have become the building blocks used to create walls of resistance. It is important to understand the difference between an excuse and a reason. Understand an excuse is not logical. You actually have to have a reason before you create the excuse. So why not stop at the reason? Or follow the reason up with a coherent action, not an irrational one.

Now let's eliminate the excuse process!

Define excuse and reason...

_____

_____

_____

_____

_____

One of the easiest ways to eliminate excuses is to educate yourself on why you're making them.

YOUR STEPS TO ELIMINATE EXCUSES

CREATE FOUR DIFFERENT WAYS YOU WILL ELIMINATE EXCUSES.

The root of a lot of excuses is fear. The fear of a response, a result, someone's opinion, etc. Fear is a distressing emotion. When distress is present in your mind, you will produce anxiety, mental suffering, pain, a sense of danger and apprehension.

Stop creating pathways of irrational thinking. Instead challenge the fear to produce logical thinking and create the ability to solve problems.

What I will do to eiliminate an excuse

What I will do to eiliminate an excuse

What I will do to eiliminate an excuse

What I will do to eiliminate an excuse

TRAINING YOUR MIND

Tell yourself at this moment, "Excuse making MUST come to an end. Believe in yourself. Speak it into existence!

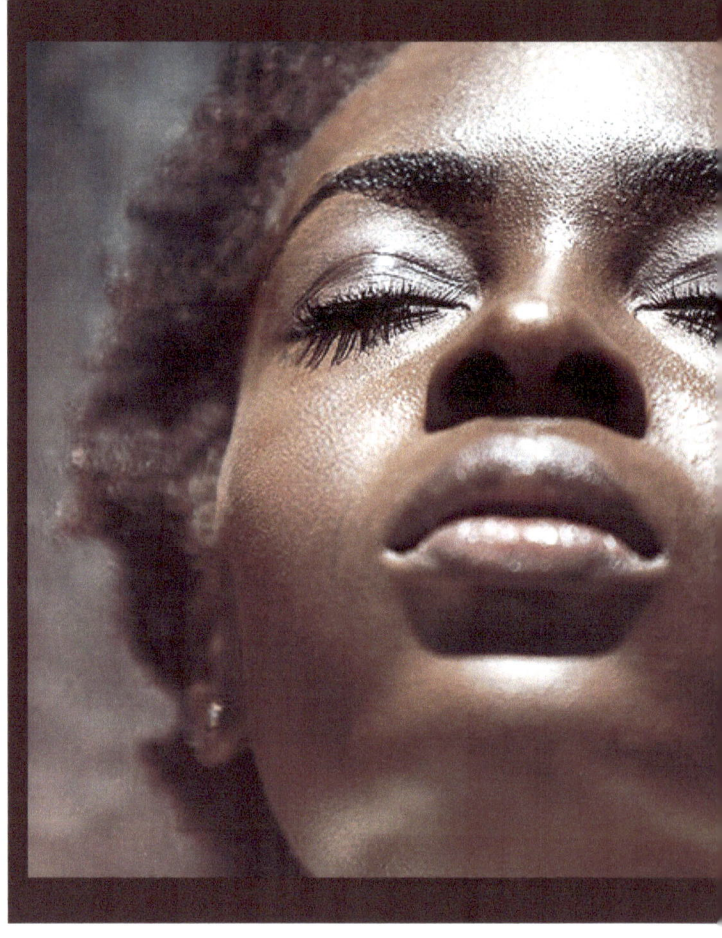

DO IT NOW!

Stop telling yourself I'll start tomorrow. You don't have tomorrow, you have today.

PLAN WITH ROOM FOR CHANGE

Too often we allow an excuse to creep in when things don't go as we planned. Prepare your mind that the unexpected will happen and you won't need to create an excuse.

STOP WORRYING ABOUT WHAT OTHER PEOPLE THINK

Learn to validate yourself. Constructive feedback is good for growth, however everyone's opinion isn't constructive, sometimes it's destructive.

BE READY TO OVERCOME DIFFICULTIES

Stop telling yourself something is too hard. Stop telling yourself no one will give you the support/help you need. You are a god. You have the ability to overcome obstacles and create what you need.

CREATE THE TIME YOU NEED

Time management is a learned skill. You must also learn how to prioritize the things in your life. Determine what's necessary and what isn't. Get rid of what isn't and place yourself in the space of productivity.

FREEDOM IN FORGIVENESS

Freedom- "Excemption from external control, interference, regulation etc. The power to determine action without restraint."

As we are beginning to understand what forgiveness actually means we must also understand it is a process. It may not happen overnight. The key is to remain focused on the end goal and be patient. Remember, this is a process.

Before you begin to read the steps in this module, I want you to first take a deep breath and clear your mind as much as you can. Remove all distractions. Turn on some relaxing music. Make some herbal tea, diffuse some essential oils, or take a nice relaxing Heal Thy Life milk bath. Do whatever you need to create your quiet, peaceful space.

THREE-STEP PROCESS

Before beginning any module, you must complete the Three-Step Process. This process is to help you enter into the state of being for healing.

STEP ONE...

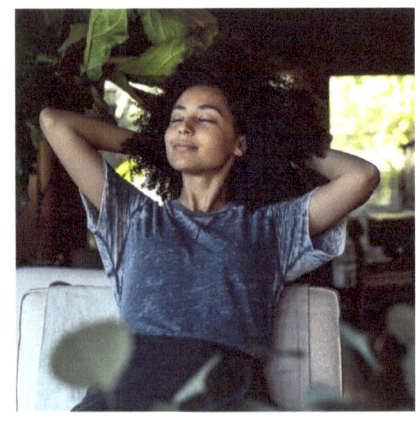

Settle into a comfortable place and breathe mindfully. Rest for two to three minutes. You should begin to feel relaxed.

STEP TWO...

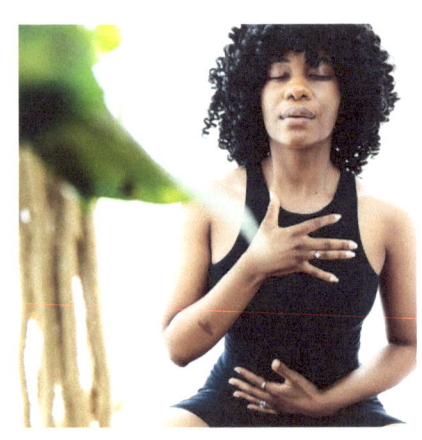

Pick an area of your body to focus on for another two to three minutes. (forehead, toes, lips, hands, etc.) Keep controlling your breathing.

STEP THREE...

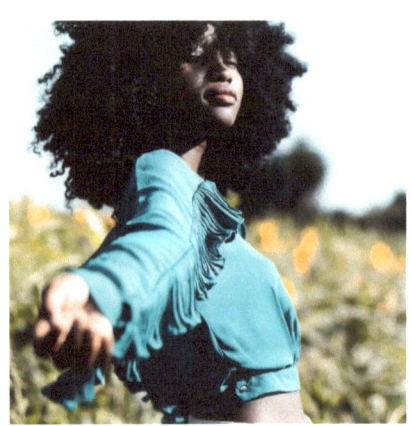

Say to yourself,
I am ready to heal.
I am ready to grow.
I am ready to become my best self!

YOUR
EMPOWERMENT
WOMEN IN HISTORY

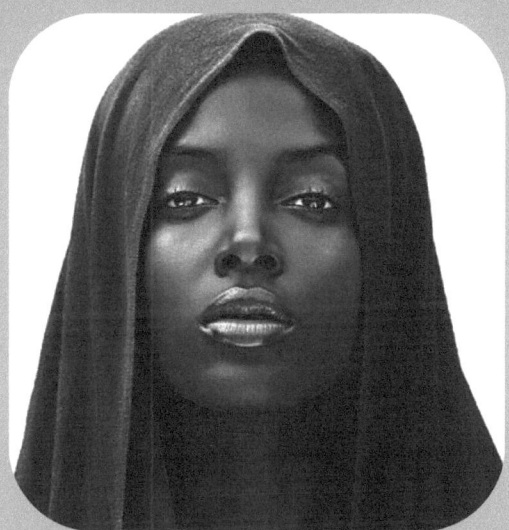

I was restored by Christ. Delivered from demonic oppression. I became one of Jesus' disciples and the head of his financial ministry. I sat at his feet washing them with expensive oil. I became his wife and bore him two children. I AM MARY OF MAGDALENE!

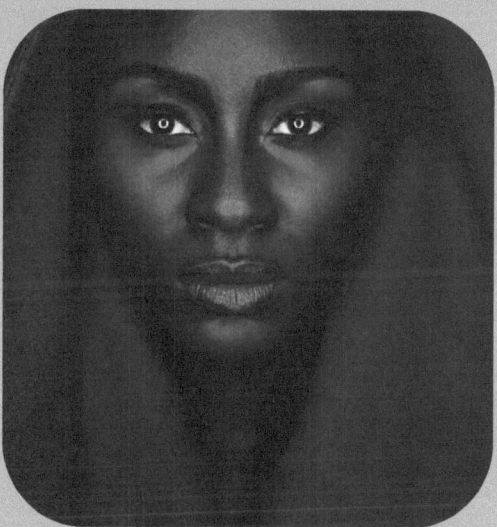

I am a strong black woman who believes in God. My faith showed I was the wife God wanted me to be to my husband so he could do what God instructed him to do. My strength comforted his. I AM THE WIFE OF MOSES, ZIPPORAH!

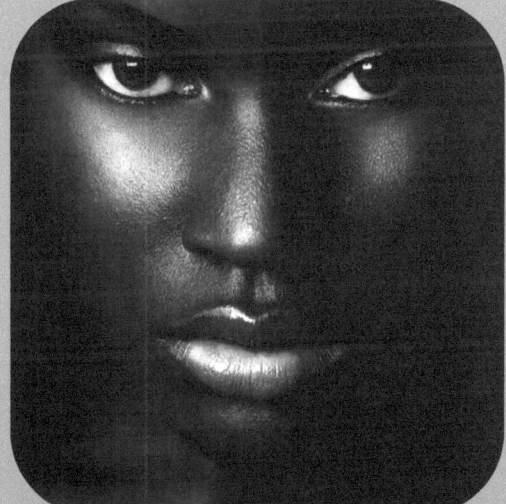

Through me you learn why a woman should never be left unprotected. I am not the downfall of man, I am the birth of his beginning. I AM MOTHER EVE!

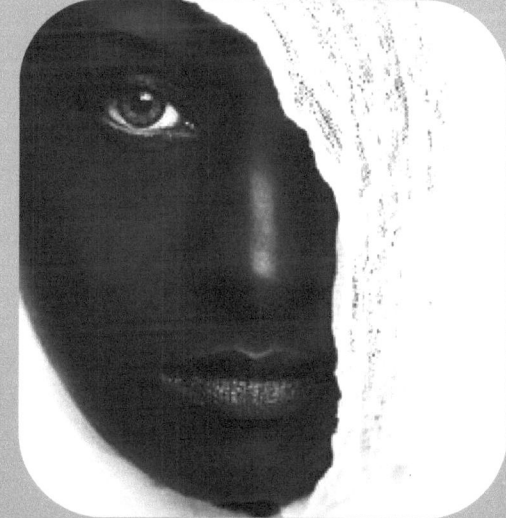

I defended Prophet Muhammad (PBUH) with my life. When he looked to his left or to his right, he saw me slaying the enemy! I am God's soldier, I AM NUSAYBAH!

THE JOURNEY OF FAITH

Walking life's journey isn't an easy task, but it's a mission you were born equipped to win. Someone told us that when we see one set of footprints in our life's journey that means God didn't leave us, but at that time He was carrying us.

I say that one set of footprints is when we become one with our Creator. We submitted to His will, we became obedient to His desires, and we allowed the God in us to be awakened and rise to its purpose.

Walk with the power of God. Have faith that moves mountains and receive the rewards on the other side.

Write how you will have faith larger than the size of a mustard seed.

_____

_____

_____

_____

_____

Faith is the key that will free you from your burdens. Faith is the seed worthy of planting into your soul. Nurture that seed with belief, water it with truth, and secure it with obedience to God.

THE FIRST THREE STEPS

There are nine steps in the Freedom in Forgiveness Process. These steps have broken up into three phases. You will have worksheets to follow each phase.

STEP ONE: BEGIN THE PROCESS

01

Write down a list of the morals and values that you have right now. Think of the things you really believe in or those things that directly influence how you function on a day-to-day basis. Take your time with this step. you may experience pain and some discomfort when you begin to connect this learned behavior with whom you've learned it from.

STEP TWO: EMBRACE SELF-ACCEPTANCE

02

You have to embrace and accept what you have done. Allow yourself to submit to this process to release yourself from the pain of what you have done to yourself. Self-guilt is a pain we have all carried. It's dangerous information that has been fed to your subconscious mind.

STEP THREE: IT HAPPENED IN THE PAST

03

In this step you need to define the phrase "It happened in the past". We are to learn from negative experiences, not be burdened by them. We have to allow healing to take place and stop punishing ourselves. God didn't create us to punish us.

NOTES

MINDFUL MEDITATION

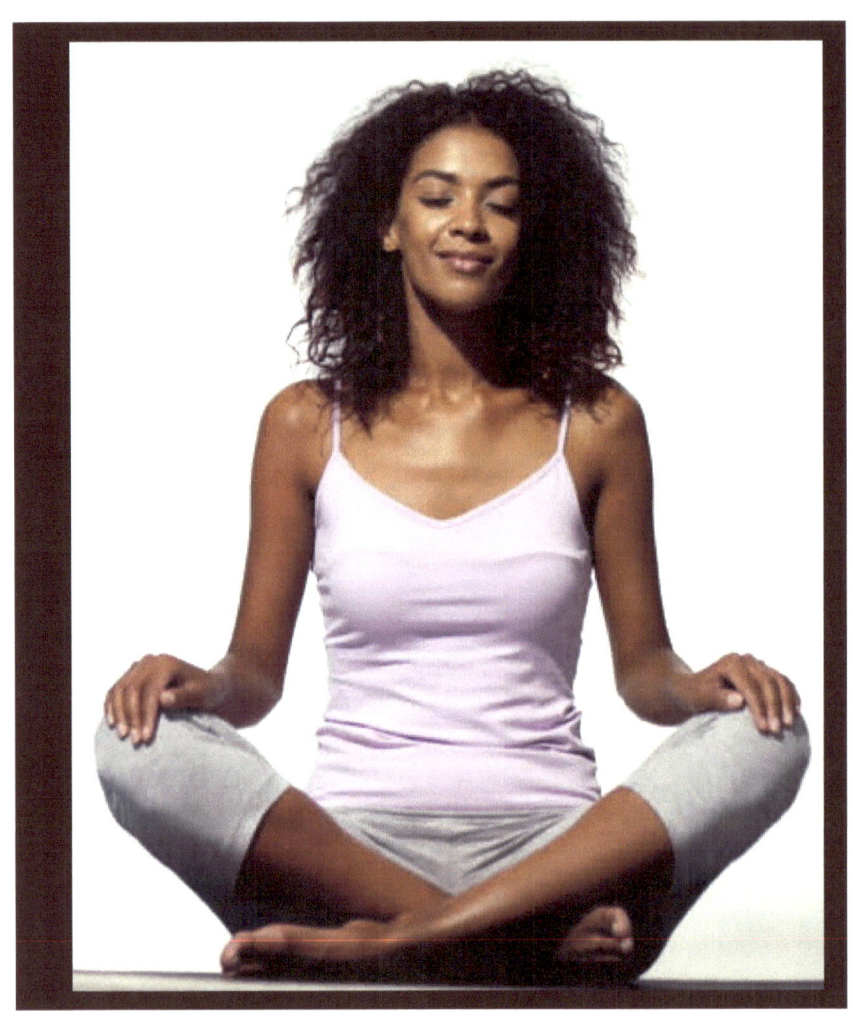

At this moment you are focusing on moving forward, embracing change and improving your outlook on life.

Step 2 is not meant to be a long process. We have to learn how to forgive and let go quickly.

Take a deep breath and create your made up mind. Tell yourself, "I exist in the present. I release the past." Believe those words, accept that is your reality and move on.

<u>*Say this affirmation to yourself*</u>
I am in the present moment
I exist right now
I am focused
I am disciplined
I am in control of my life
I am positive motion
I am a new reality

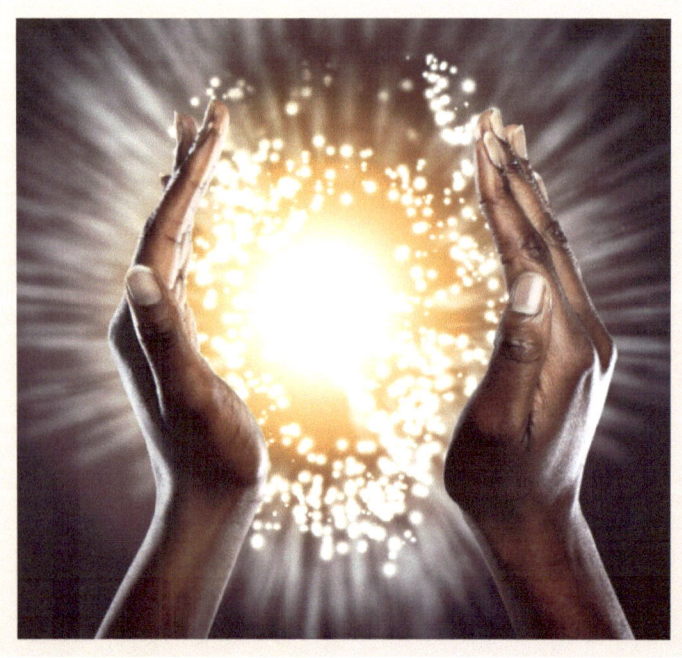

MINDFUL MEDITATION PART 2

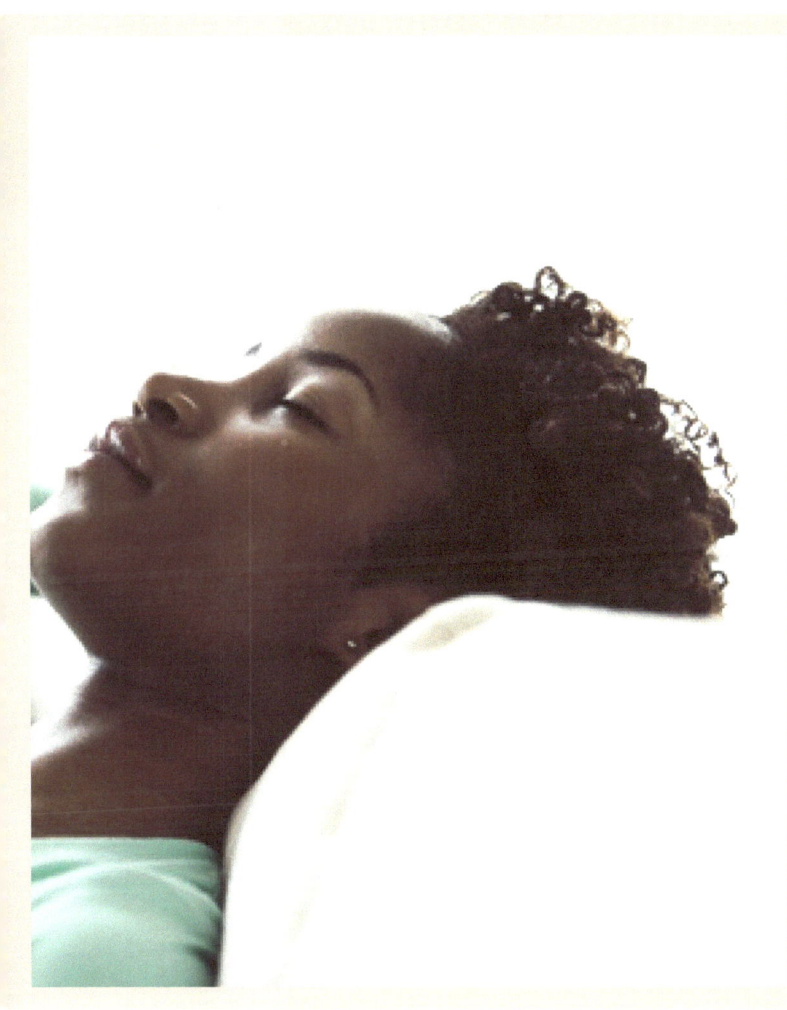

You can not change what has happened in the past. There is something you can do! You can learn from it and release yourself from the emotions attached to past events or behaviors. You have the power to do so. Don't allow a past experience to determine the outcome of your life.

Healing from a negative experience can be just as simple as removing the blame from yourself. Tell yourself it was not your fault. If it was your fault, tell yourself you have learned to do better.

STOP PUNISHING YOURSELF with thoughts of self-destruction. Focus on the incredible future you are about to walk into.

Say this affirmation to yourself
I am peaceful
I am balanced
I am calm

I am positive energy
I am centered
I am connected to all that is
I feed off of my Creator and the Universe
I am one

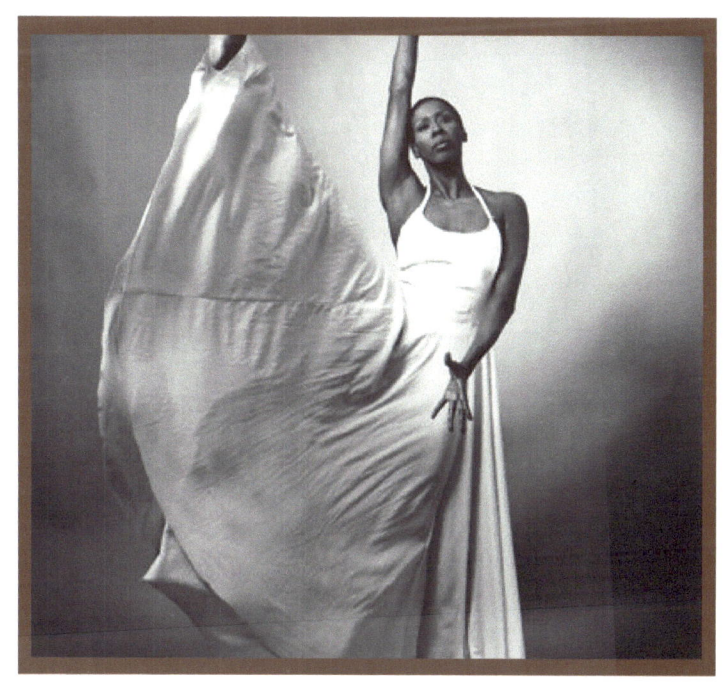

THE NEXT THREE STEPS

The next three steps deal with pain, discomfort and hate. You WILL need to take a break during these steps. Do not try to complete these steps in a day or two. Take your time. Have pleasurable thoughts ready for activation. Be patient and kind to yourself.

STEP FOUR: PAIN

The wrong type of pain restricts us. You must believe you have the power to release the negative energy that is holding you captive. You are in the process of reprogramming your thinking and becoming in tune with your inner power. Believe that.

STEP FIVE: DISCOMFORT AND HATE

If you have experienced pain, you have felt discomfort and possibly hate, which is ok. Discomfort should put us in a productive state seeking ease. It should be recognized as motivation. We are to hate what God hates. Ex. God hates sin, not the sinner.

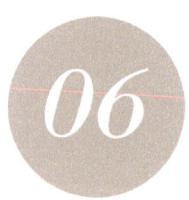

STEP SIX: DETERMINE WHAT YOU WANT

Determine what you want to release. You may want to release shame, guilt, blame, etc. Take the time to understand what you want. Connect with your Creator for His strength and guidance. Be convicted in your decision.

NOTES

IDENTIFY

Identify one experience of pain you carry. (ONLY ONE) You don't want to overwhelm yourself. While identifying this experience, be sure to identify the emotions attached to the experience.

WHAT IS ONE OF YOUR EXPERIENCES OF PAIN?

_____

_____

_____

_____

_____

_____

WHAT ARE THE EMOTIONS CONNECTED TO THIS EXPERIENCE?

_____

_____

_____

_____

_____

DISCOMFORT AND HATE

Learn to love yourself and assist God in your healing process.

WHAT PURPOSE DID PAIN SERVE IN YOUR LIFE? (ONE EXAMPLE)

_____

_____

WHEN DID DISCOMFORT MOTIVATE YOU TO BE PRODUCTIVE?

_____

_____

WHAT IS AN EXAMPLE OF HATING WHAT GOD HATES?

_____

_____

WHAT IS ONE MOMENT IN YOUR LIFE YOU WERE NOT IN CONTROL OF YOUR EMOTIONS?

_____

_____

CONFRONT AND CONFESS

In this exercise you will list times you were in control of your emotions and times when you were not. List events that are both past and present. Confront the events and confess them to yourself. Ask your Creator to open up the doorway to your healing. Take as many breaks as you feel are needed. This is a process that takes time.

CONTROLLED EMOTIONS   UNCONTROLLED EMOTIONS

STOP

DANCE

—

AND

SMILE

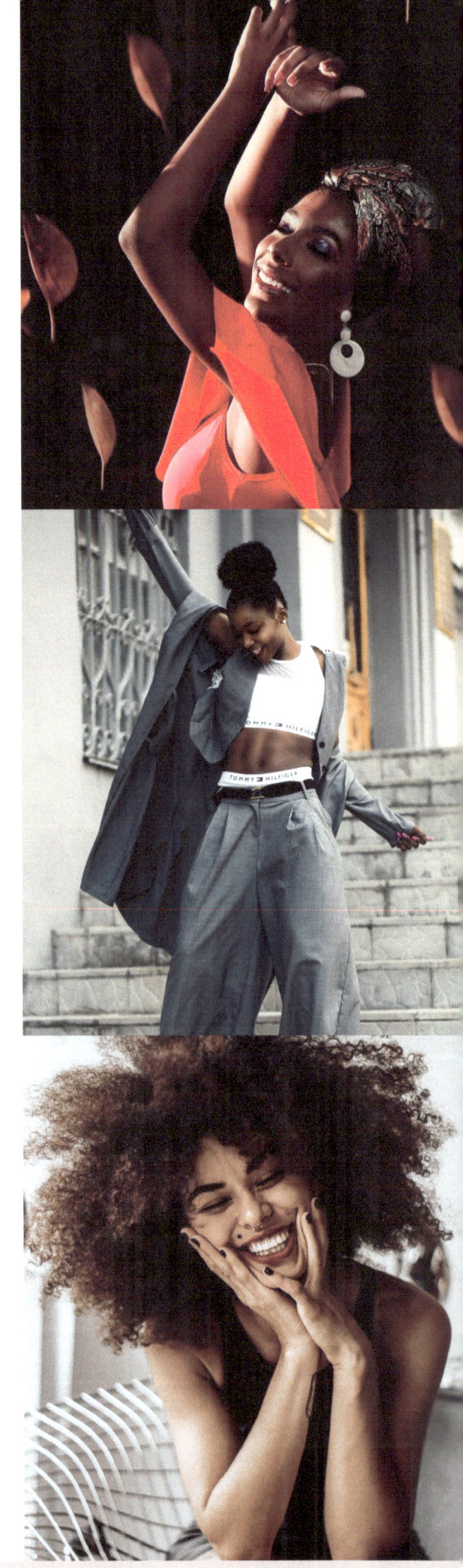

What Do You Want To Experience?

Write down what you would like to release. What are some of the things you are holding on to? Be hopeful and balanced in your capability. Connect with the core of your being to release your pain and unwanted emotions. Say aloud, "You don't belong to me anymore. I release you and no longer desire for you to be with me. From this day forth you will only exist in my past having no effect on my present and future. My past is no longer apart of my present. I live in the present."

THE LAST THREE STEPS

Time to reward yourself! You are becoming a better you. Get excited!

07 STEP SEVEN: REWARD YOURSELF

Knowing that you have completed the previous steps reassures you that you can complete the Freedom in Forgiveness process. Repeat it as many times as necessary until there is no longer a need for it. You are writing your history in advance! CELEBRATE!

08 STEP EIGHT: SELF-LOVE

Retrain your thinking to love yourself. You have just completed seven steps. That is proof that you love yourself. Continue to demonstrate your love of self by continuing the process needed to better yourself.

09 STEP NINE: CLAIM THE NEW AND IMPROVED YOU

Embrace who you are becoming. Thank God, thank yourself, and walk in your new found light.

NOTES

CREATE YOUR REWARD SYSTEM

List different ways to reward yourself. Note: DO NOT use food as a reward.

REWARD ONE

REWARD TWO

REWARD THREE

REWARD FOUR

•WANTED•

FREEDOM

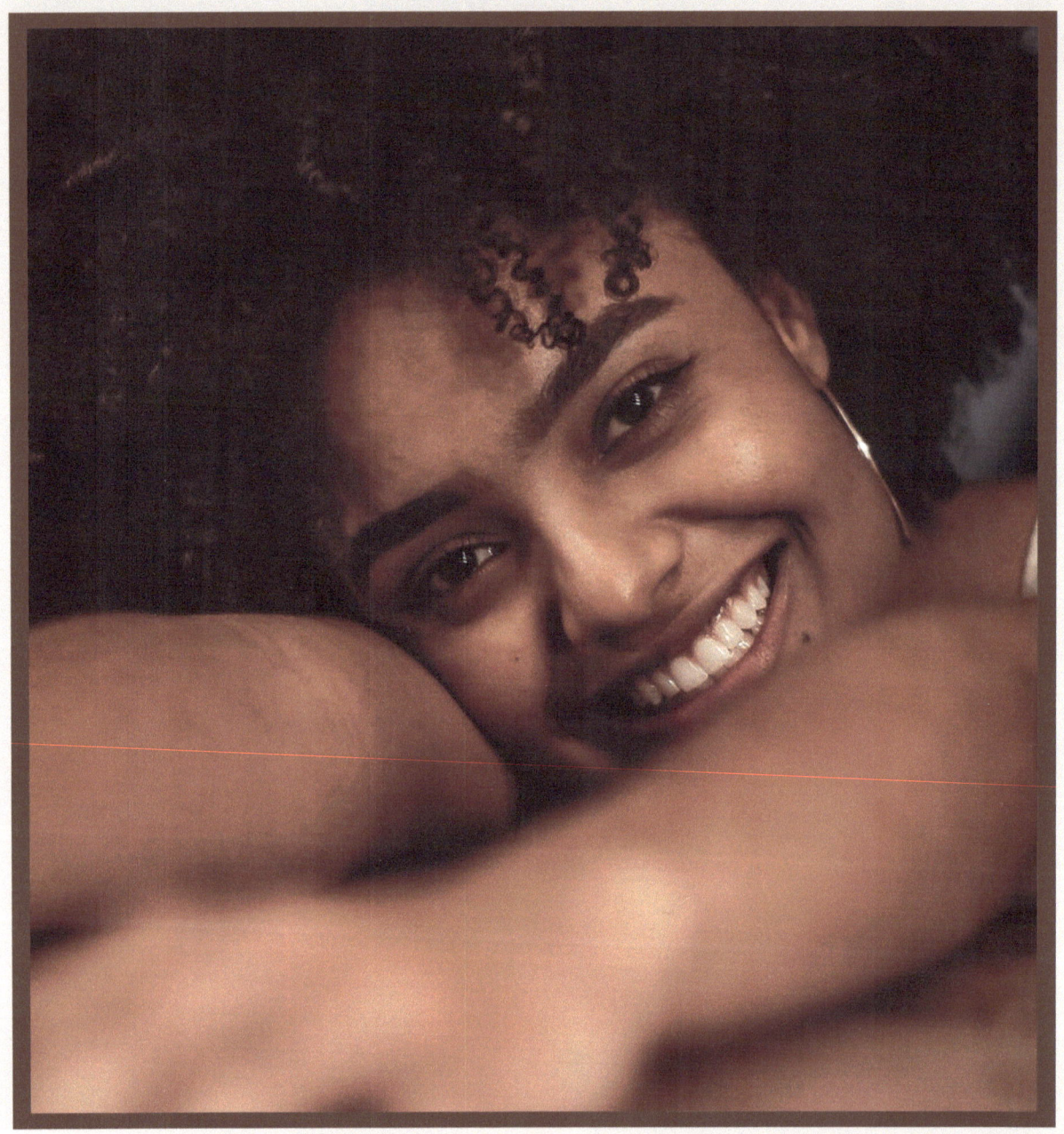

REWARD: HAPPINESS

GOD CHOSE ME

Letter To Self

DEAR SELF,

I love you!

And this is why...

My own best friend,

(sign your name)

P.S. I will never go back to my old way of thinking.

PLACE A PICTURE OF THE NEW AND IMPROVED YOU BELOW

I'm Growing!

EMOTION = ENERGY IN MOTION

Did you know that most of our emotions are learned behavior? Just like with colors, we have primary emotions and secondary emotions. Primary emotions are what we are born with. They are apart of our nature and usually what we feel first in a situation. Secondary emotions build off of the primary, being influenced by our experiences. As a result, they are considered to be learned behaviors. For example, a person has to feel sadness before they experience depression. You are angry before you become enraged.

Our primary emotions are anger, happiness, fear and sadness. Secondary emotions can be shame, envy, jealousy, frustration, hate, etc. It is important to note that doubt, according to The Honorable Min. Louis Farrakhan, is often considered an emotion but it is not; instead it is actually a state of mind. It is good to know the difference between a state of mind and an emotion and how one affects the other.

THREE-STEP PROCESS

Before beginning any module, you must complete the three step process. This process is to help you enter into the state of being for healing.

STEP ONE...

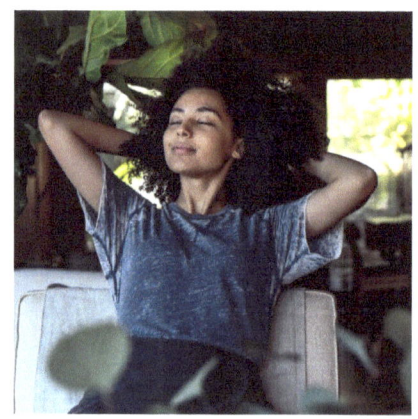

Settle into a comfortable place and breathe mindfully. Rest for two to three minutes. You should begin to feel relaxed.

STEP TWO...

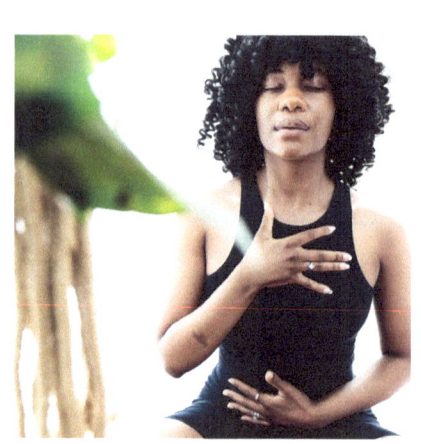

Pick an area of your body to focus on for another two to three minutes (forehead, toes, lips, hands, etc.). Keep controlling your breathing.

STEP THREE...

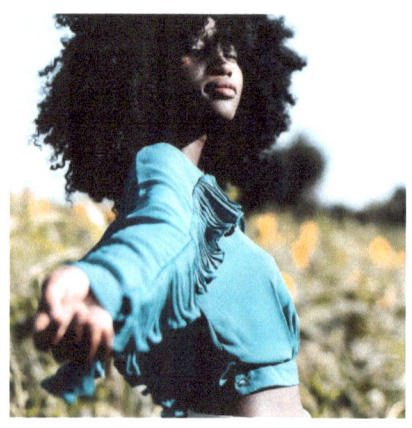

Say to yourself,
I am ready to heal.
I am ready to grow.
I am ready to become my best self!

YOUR EMPOWERMENT

WOMEN IN HISTORY

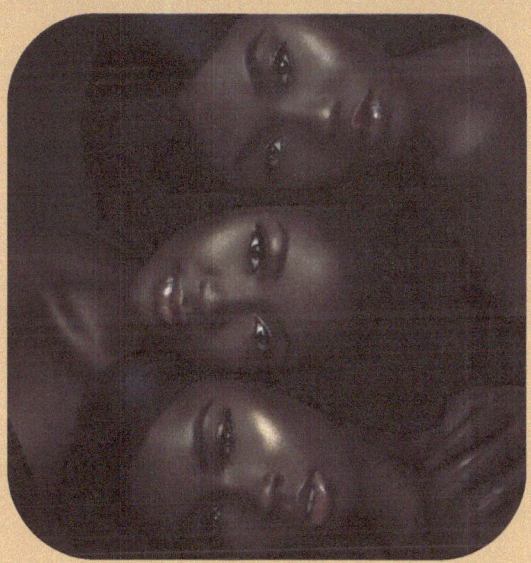

We are women of God! We are faithful, loyal, virtuous and strong. We are clothed with dignity and speak with wisdom. WE ARE THE WOMEN OF PROVERBS 31!

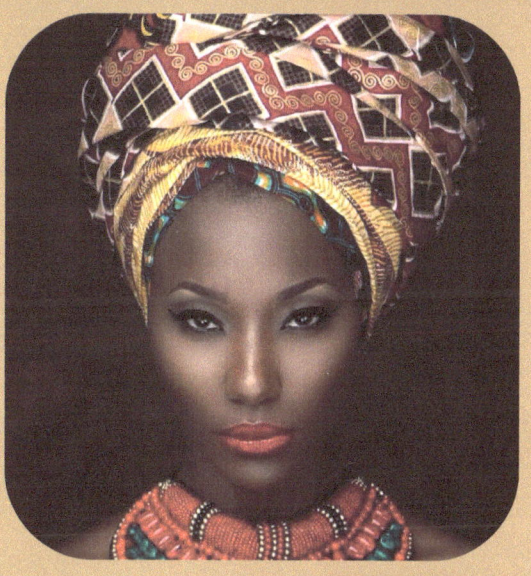

I believed in one God! I reigned during the wealthiest period of Ancient Egyptian history. I was a woman of beauty and power. I AM QUEEN NERFERTITI.

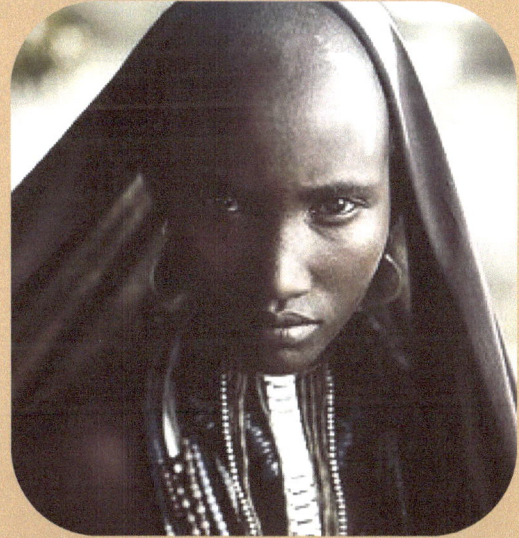

I endured great humiliation and rejection. I had great influences over African affairs. I was my son's pillar of strength. I AM THE MOTHER OF SHAKA ZULU, I AM QUEEN NANDI!

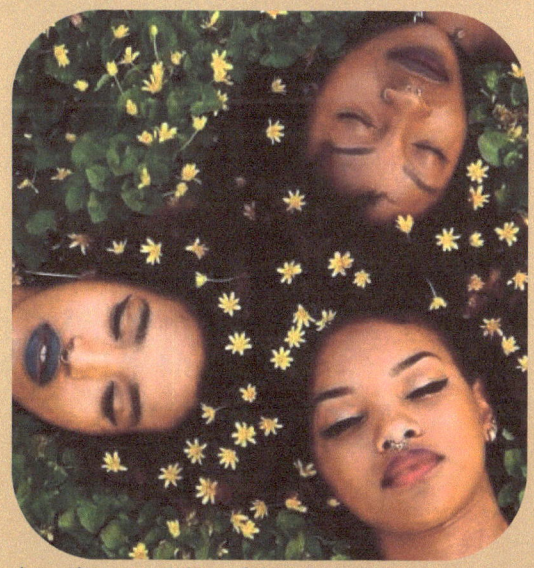

We inspire positive thinking. We empower one another. We lift, support, protect and lean on each other. WE ARE MOTHER NATURE'S HEALING CIRCLE!

ENERGY IN MOTION

The word emotion comes from the Latin term *emovere*, which means 'moving'. Our emotions are energetic vibrations moving through our bodies and around the outside of our bodies. Emotions are contagious. Just think about it. How many times have you witnessed your mood affect others? How many times have other people's moods affected yours? A happy person carries positive energetic forces giving them the ability to bring up another person's tone. Similarly, an angry person carries the energetic force to bring the mood down in someone.

When was a time someone's emotions affected yours?

_____

_____

_____

_____

_____

I am the peace during times of difficulty.

ARE MY EMOTIONS CONTROLLING ME?

We have to learn how to control our emotions. You become irrational when your thoughts and behaviors are controlling you. You explode and say things you shouldn't say or you do things you shouldn't do.

WHEN WAS A TIME YOU ALLOWED YOUR EMOTIONS TO TAKE CONTROL OF YOU?

OUR BODIES RESPOND TO
STRESSFUL EMOTIONS AS IF
THEY'RE IN A STATE OF
EMERGENCY!

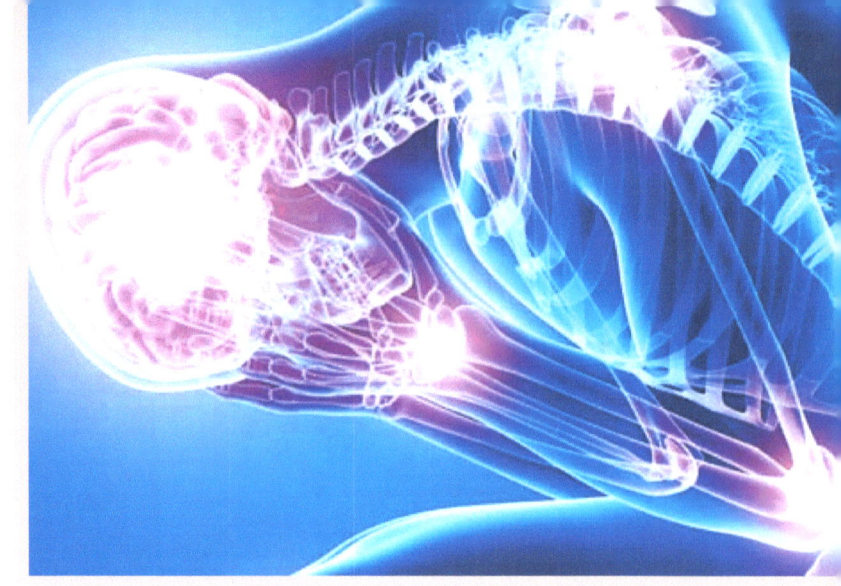

AVOID THE SHUT DOWN

ATTACK

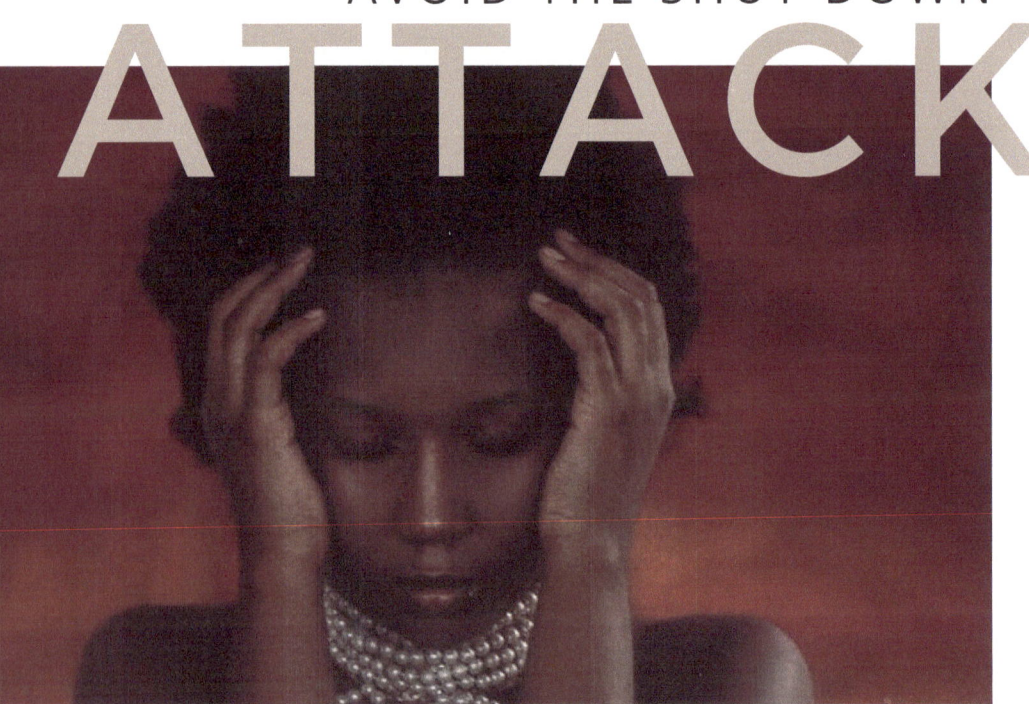

STRESSFUL
EMOTIONS ARE
IDENTIFIED IN OUR
BODIES AS A THREAT
WHICH ACTIVATES
OUR IMMUNE
SYSTEM.

EMOTIONS CAN OVERWHELM
OUR RATIONAL THOUGHTS,
LEADING TO OUR BODILY
FUNCTIONS SHUTTING
DOWN.

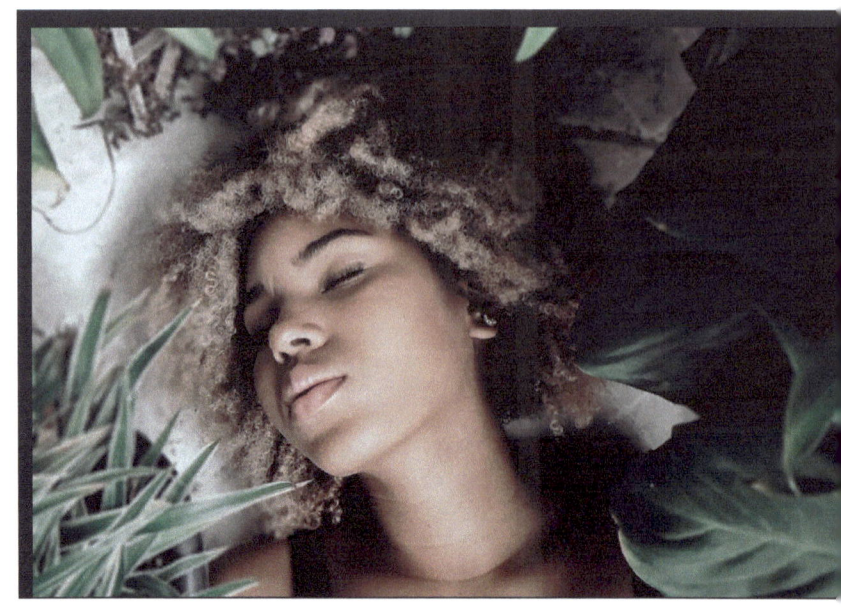

RECOGNIZE THE SHUT DOWN

Quiet your mind and answer the following questions.

HAVE YOU EVER GOTTEN SO ANGRY THAT YOU FOUND YOURSELF AT A LOSS FOR WORDS? IF SO, WRITE AN APOLOGY TO YOURSELF.

_____

_____

HAVE YOU EVER GOTTEN SO SAD YOU DIDN'T WANT TO EAT? IF SO, WRITE AN APOLOGY TO YOURSELF.

_____

_____

HAVE YOU EVER SEEN A CHILD SO AFRAID THAT THEY USED THE BATHROOM ON THEMSELVES? IF SO, UNDERSTAND THAT CAN HAPPEN TO YOU TOO.

_____

_____

CAN YOU GIVE AN EXAMPLE OF WHEN YOU WERE OVERWHELMED WITH EMOTIONS?

_____

_____

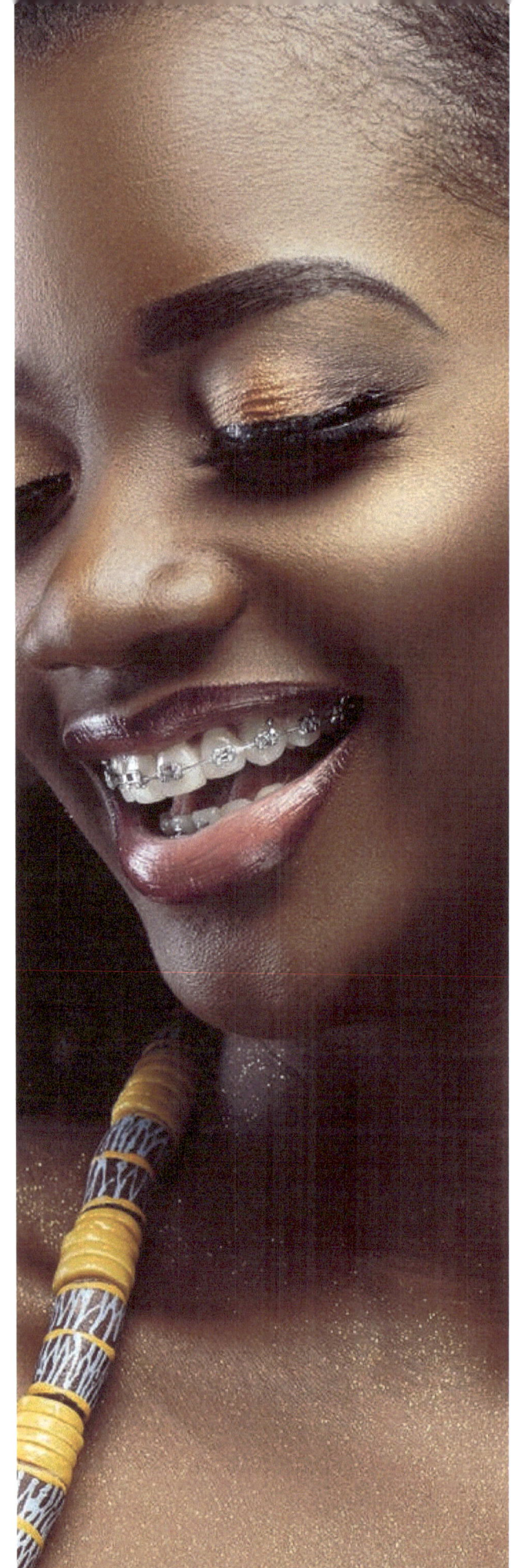

HEALING BEGINS IN THE MIND

Make your mind your best asset, not your worst enemy!

BELIEF

Believe your healing is real. Believe you have the power to heal. What you believe influences how your body responds. Eliminate what others believe and accept what you believe.

GRATITUDE

Being grateful heals the mind and helps to calm your soul. Before you go to bed at night, think of all the things you are grateful for from that day.

FEEL IT

Feelings and thoughts are connected but separate. Get in tune with the way you feel so you can control the thoughts you manifest. Give yourself time to connect with your feelings. Be patient, this may take some time.

MIXED EMOTIONS

Mixed emotions are a combination of emotions that can be expressed simultaneously or one after the other. Mixed emotions are common to a certain degree and can be normal. For example, waiting on a new job or the birth of a child can produce anxiety, fear and excitement. That's normal.

However, mixed emotions become dangerous when the wrong ingredients are put together. An example is when self-esteem is mixed with entitlement, which can lead to narcissism. Anxiety can be produced by fear combined with excitement because of anticipation. But fear mixed with anger can produce the type of anxiety that causes mental illness or disease to set up in the body.

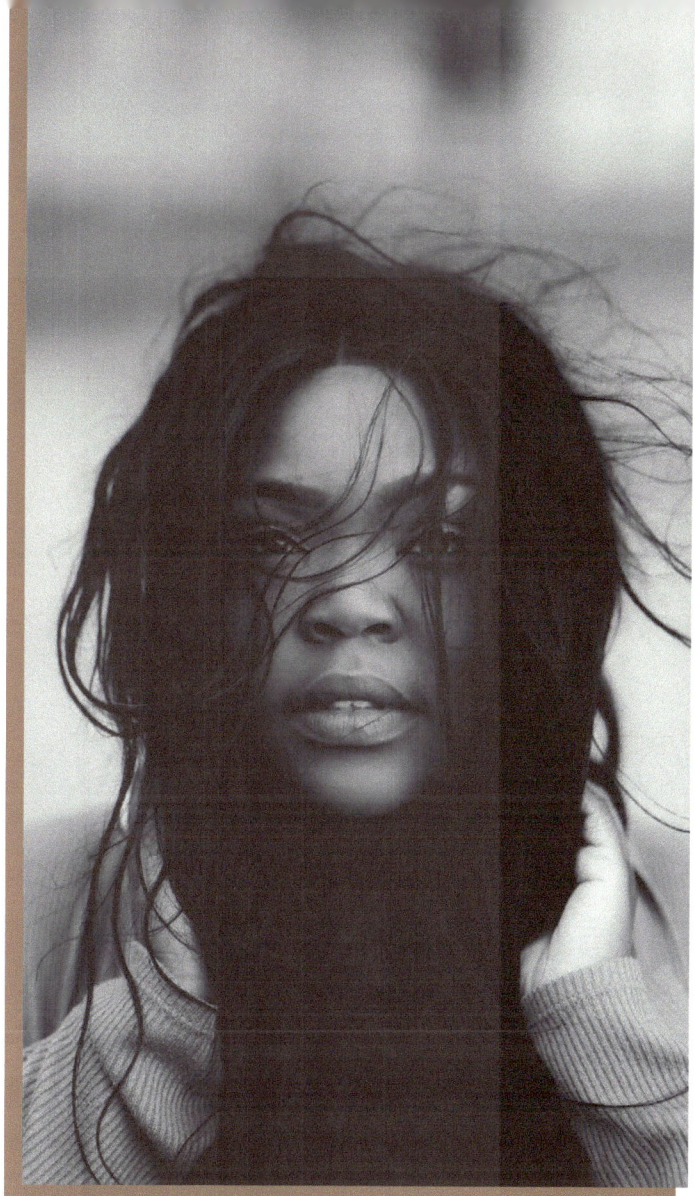

REFLECTION

RELEASE YOUR TEARS

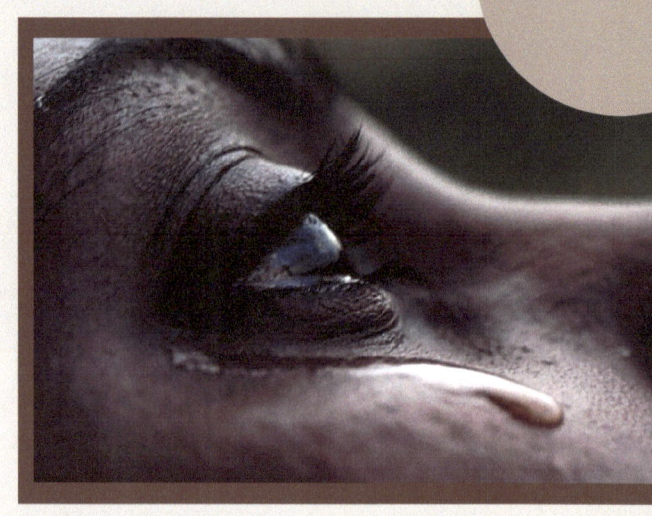

Crying is not weak. Stop holding your tears back even in cases where you are "waiting on the right time to release".

"Emotional tears were found to contain high levels of the hormones and neurotransmitters associated with stress."
-Dr. Willam Frey

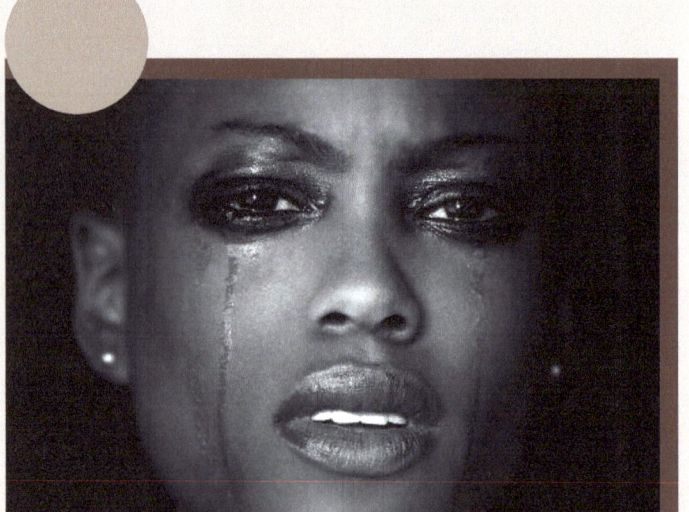

The purpose of emotional crying is to remove stressful chemicals from the body.

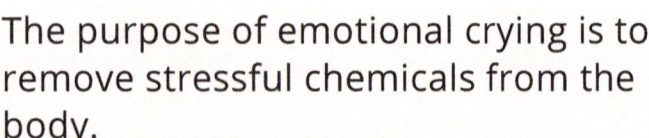

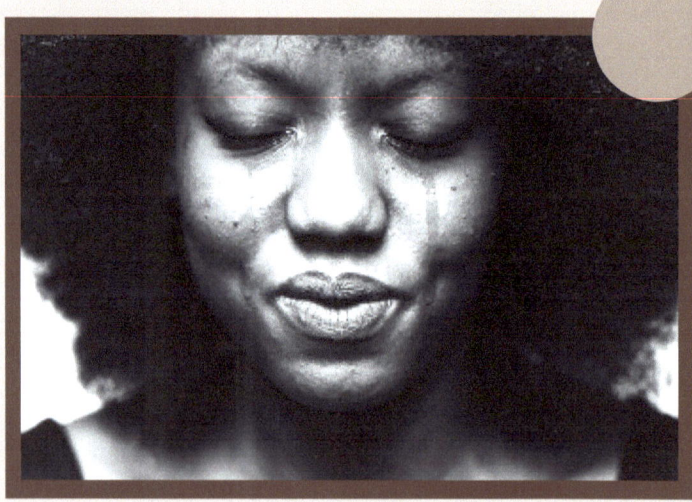

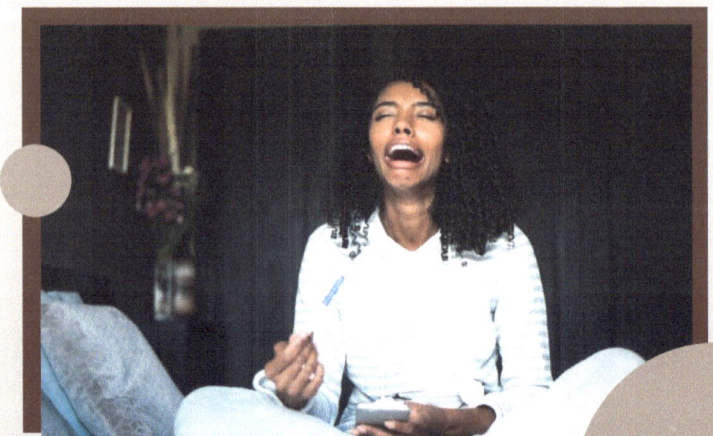

Holding back tears leaves the body prone to anxiety, a weakened immune system, impaired memory, and poor digestion.

Boost Your Immune System

Gratitude

If you desire the organs of your body to operate at a high level of frequency, all you have to do is express gratitude. Doctors have proven that the feelings of gratitude boost immunity, lower blood pressure and speed up healing.

Fall in love with who you are

Falling in love raises levels of nerve growth factor, improves memory, triggers the growth of new brain cells, and produces a calming effect on the body and the mind. LOVE IS LIFE!

Laugh

Laughter creates high mood boosting beta-endorphins in the body, aids in sleep, cellular repair, and reduces levels of stress! Laughter has even been found to reduce the risk of a heart attack! Laughing strengthens the lungs and assists with healing the mind.

Write What You Are Grateful For

Take a deep breath and relax your mind. Let gratitude flow through your body as it is expressed through the pen.

A Promise of Love To Self

Dear self,

I promise to love you!

Here are the ways I will love myself...

My own love,

(sign your name)

P.S. I will never mistreat myself again.

MY LAUGHTER

Place a picture of you laughing below. Only you! You deserve this moment of healing. It's all about you!

SAY CHEESE

MAKING YOUR BREAKING POINT YOUR BREAKTHROUGH

A person's breaking point can be defined as the moment they break down or give way. At this point, the stress in life has built up so much that things in the individual's life begin to fall apart. The beauty of this, is that in the process, you have the ability to turn it around. The body gives us warning signs in advance.

When you feel yourself beginning to break, take a proactive stance and start looking for a solution. You can also create the answers to your problems in advance. This will help you turn your breakdown into a breakthrough. Become determined. Use the intensity of your emotions to create your win. You DON'T have to cross your breaking point! And, in the case that you do, you have what it takes to get through it.

THREE-STEP PROCESS

Before beginning any module, you must complete the three step process. This process is to help you enter into the state of being for healing.

STEP ONE...

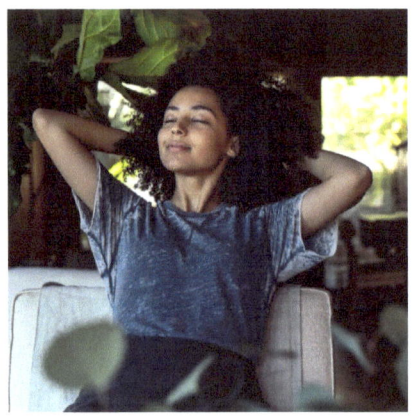

Settle into a comfortable place and breathe mindfully. Rest for two to three minutes. You should begin to feel relaxed.

STEP TWO...

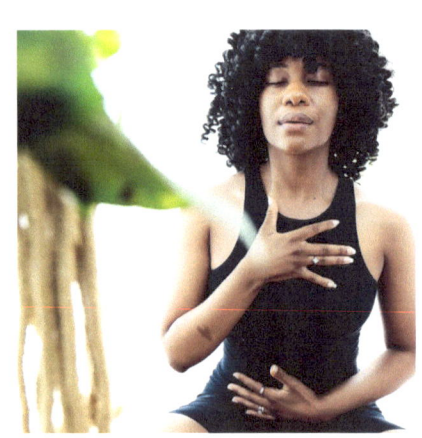

Pick an area of your body to focus on for another two to three minutes (forehead, toes, lips, hands, etc.). Keep controlling your breathing.

STEP THREE...

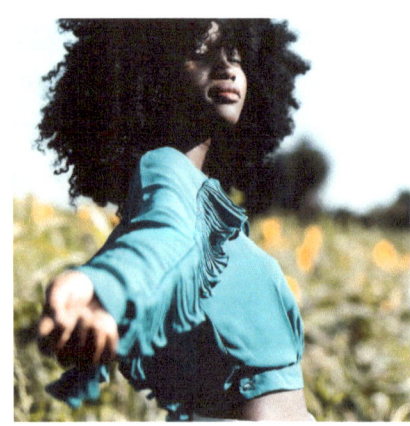

Say to yourself,
I am ready to heal.
I am ready to grow.
I am ready to become my best self!

YOUR
EMPOWERMENT
WOMEN IN HISTORY

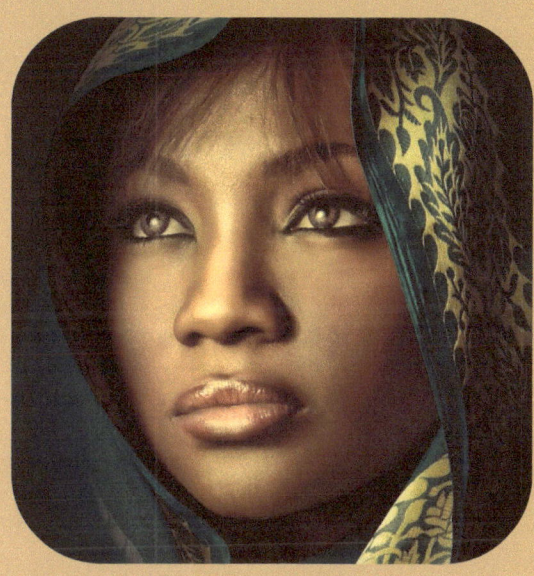

Many discriminated against me, but God loved me. Many didn't see my worth, but God placed me in the lineage of Jesus. I am a loyal companion and a comforter. I am a woman of my word. I AM THE BIBLICAL RUTH!

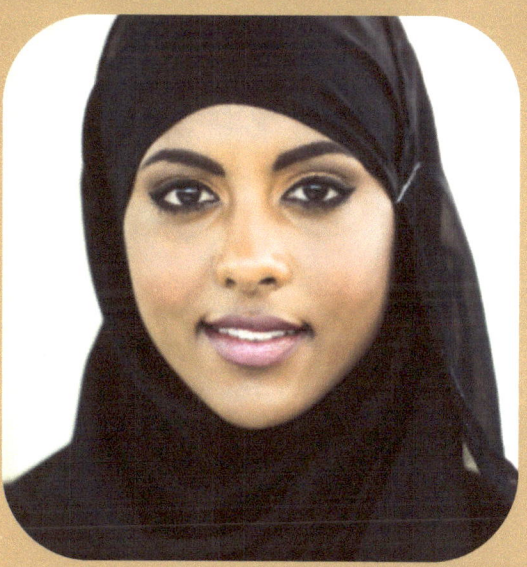

I was the daughter who reflected my father's character. I am a truthful and modest woman. I have suffered the loss of many. I remained strong and patient. I am the daughter of Prophet Muhammad (PBUH), I AM FATIMA!

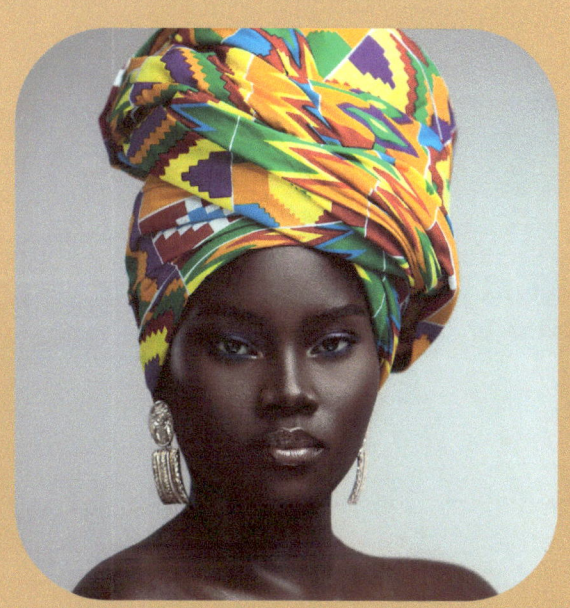

I was kidnapped from Ghana and forced into slavery in Jamaica. I escaped the misery of slavery and freed 800 slaves. I defeated the British on several occasions.   I AM QUEEN NANNY!

Phase Four

BE CURIOUS AND COURAGEOUS

You deserve to live life to the fullest. Seek what exists outside of your everyday activities. Become courageous enough to go out and get it. Tell yourself you will no longer live a life that's falling apart. You will take charge of your life. You are in control with God's permission.

Surrender yourself to your Creator. Build your faith. Trust Him. When you feel you're nearing or at a breakdown, surround yourself with God. Let everything else go! That moment to breathe creates a clear mind letting you see what and who belongs in your life. It also allows you to see what and who doesn't belong.

WHEN I FEEL OVERWHELMING PRESSURE COMING ON, THESE ARE THE WORDS I WILL SAY TO RELEASE:

_____

_____

_____

_____

_____

You have the ultimate power!
Use your power of choice!

IDENTIFY THE BREAKDOWN

In the space provided, write down the signs you identify with your having a breakdown. Be sure to include signs that show you're approaching a breakdown.

WHAT DOES ANXIETY FEEL LIKE TO YOU?

WHAT DO YOUR MOOD SWINGS FEEL LIKE?

WHAT DOES YOU BEING OVERWHELMED FEEL LIKE?

WHEN DO YOU HAVE DIFFICULTY FOCUSING?

HAVE YOU EXPERIENCED ANY UNEXPLAINED ACHES AND PAINS? DO YOU CONTINUOUSLY FEEL EMOTIONALLY DRAINED AND PHYSICALLY EXHAUSTED?

SOLUTION

WRITE THE NUMBER ONE ACTION YOU CAN DO TO AVOID A BREAKDOWN

CREATE YOUR STEPS TO PREVENT YOUR BREAKDOWN

THREATS TO MY COURAGE	RESPONSES TO PROTECT IT

NOTE: TO PREVENT PROCRASTINATION THIS ACTIVITY SHOULD BE COMPLETED BY A SELF-IMPOSED DATE. KEEP UP THE MOMENTUM OF YOUR HEALING PROCESS.

MY DEADLINE _____   MARK AS COMPLETE

AM I LIVING IN SURVIVAL MODE?

Many of us live very stressful lives. We grow up in communities designed to create circumstances that mold us to live in constant survival mode, which is the lowest level of existence.

Living in survival mode breaks down the cells and systems of the human body and blocks the proper usage of our emotions. It is imperative that we get out of survival mode. The proper way to do this is to first recognize who you are. Next, you must recognize how valuable you are no matter what you have been told in your life.

God poured His love into you as He shaped and molded you. Your life is meant to be in existence!

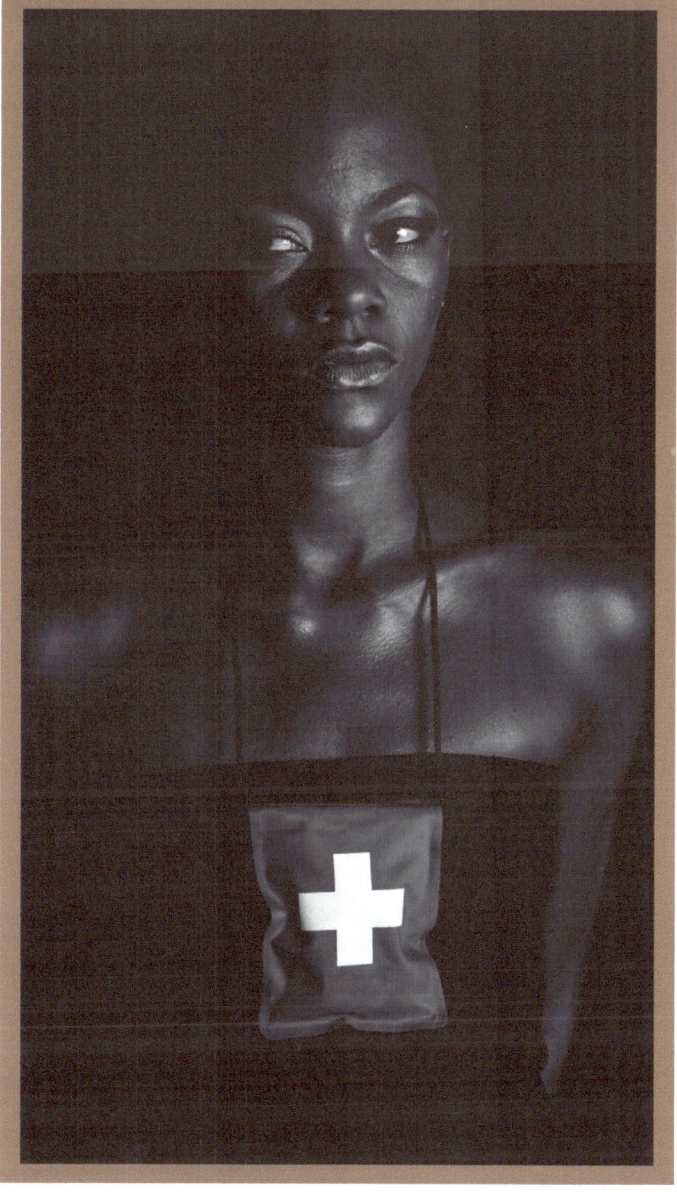

WHY AM I VALUABLE?

SURVIVAL MODE CHECKLIST

Below is a list of signs that you are living in survival mode. They are not in any particular order.

24HOURS

When your life is all about getting through the next 24hrs and the end of the week feels a long way off.

COMPLAINTS AND ROUTINES

The joy in life has been replaced with complaints and routine days.

URGENT

Everything in life is urgent. The deadline is now.

REACTION

Reaction has become your first nature and being proactive doesn't even exist as an option.

RESTLESSNESS

You don't sleep well at night because you're worried about tomorrow. Your breathing is irregular along with your heartbeat.

YOUR NEXT MEAL

All you can think about is where your next meal will come from or how you're going to pay your bills.

GET OUT OF SURVIVAL MODE

We have the ability to get out of survival mode. It is not in our nature to be in such a condition. We are gods!

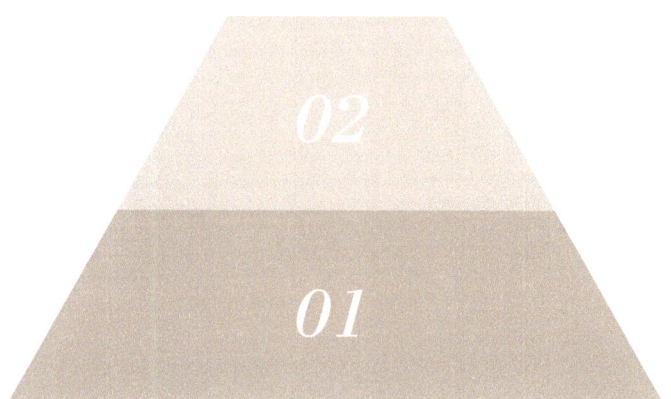

ACKNOWLEDGE YOUR REALITY

Stop denying your current reality in life. Own up to it and get out of it.

REDIFINE YOUR YOU

It doesn't matter what others have told you in life. You define who you are!

RECOGNIZE GOD TOOK A MOMENT TO CREATE YOU

Build your connection with God by building your gratitude for the life He created.

YOUR LIFE IS MEANT TO BE IN EXISTENCE

God poured His love into you. He shaped and molded you. You are not a mistake. You have worth and value. Give God the power over your life and watch how your life will change.

YOU ARE POWERFUL

Recognize who you are. Have fun in creating the new and improved you. Allow no one to take this moment away from you. You deserve it.

BE HONEST WITH YOURSELF

Being honest with yourself is the only way you can exit your current reality with healing. While you're going through this step acknowledge and assess the inner emotions you're feeling. Validate each one of them.

FINANCIAL DEPOSITS

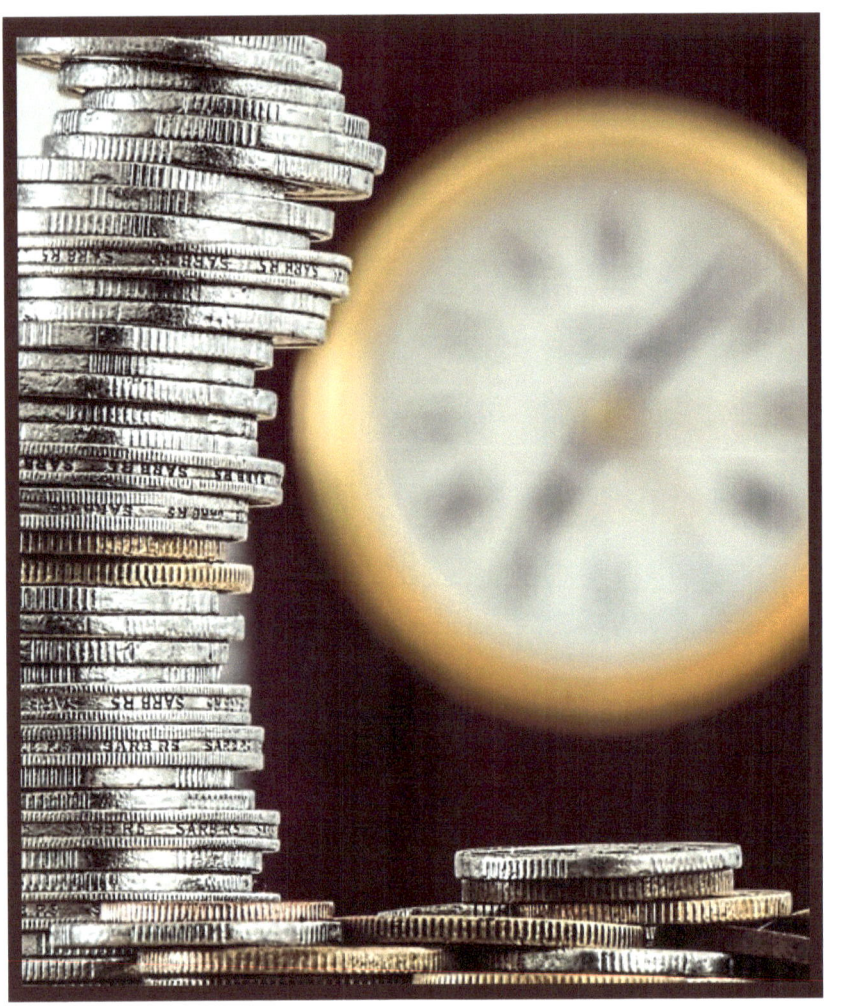

Stop over spending. If your current income doesn't allow you to make certain purchases, then don't. Instead focus on creating a way to grow your income. It is more important to place your money in areas that count. Don't sabotage yourself by creating financial burdens.

Too many of us are breaking down because of financial burdens. Take a snapshot of how much money you are spending everyday. Create a financial journal. Log in every time you spend money and track it all the way down to the penny.

Say this affirmation to yourself
I am financially free
I am in control of my life
I am inspired
I am driven
I am positive energy
I am a new reality

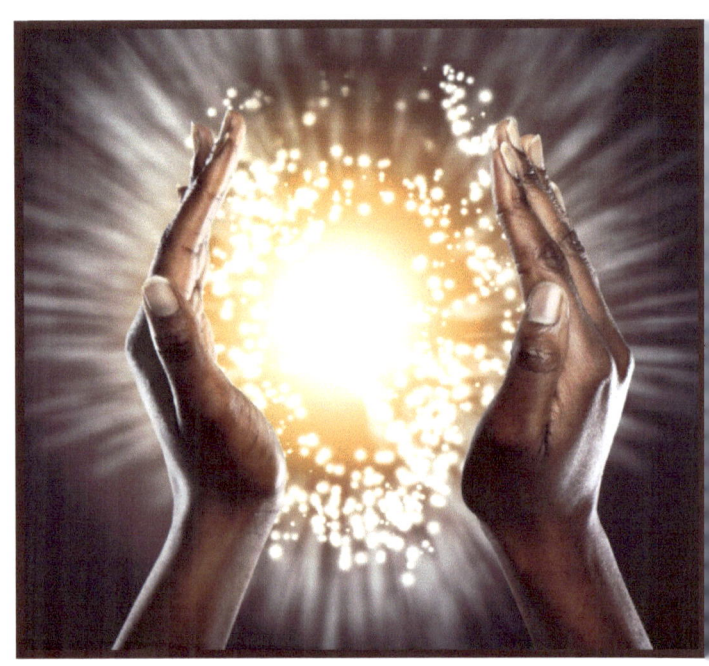

LOG WHAT YOU ARE SPENDING

Begin to log what type of spending you are doing. Look at how much money you have coming in. You can refer to page 51 of my book "The Power to Break Generational Pain" for additional guidance with this activity.

GOOD SPENDING   BAD SPENDING

GOOD SPENDING   BAD SPENDING

GOOD SPENDING   VS   BAD SPENDING

GOOD SPENDING   BAD SPENDING

GOOD SPENDING   BAD SPENDING

LOG SPIRITUAL DEPOSITS

Everything you do physically you must do spiritually. Are you depositing the bare minimum into your spirit? Are you withdrawing things that feed faithlessness? When you feel yourself nearing or at a breakdown, you only need to surround yourself with God.

FAITH DEPOSIT   FAITHLESSNESS REMOVAL

FAITH DEPOSIT   FAITHLESSNESS REMOVAL

FAITH DEPOSIT   FAITHLESSNESS REMOVAL

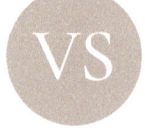

FAITH DEPOSIT   FAITHLESSNESS REMOVAL

FAITH DEPOSIT   FAITHLESSNESS REMOVAL

CREATE YOUR BREAKTHROUGH

Don't wait for what you may define as the perfect time. That time may never come. The time for action is now. You can start off with small breakthroughs en route to the big one. Recognize new ideas and thoughts that will flow through your mind. Write them down and act on them. You have to be alert and observant when creating and accepting your moment of breakthrough.

HOW CAN I BE ALERT AND OBSERVANT?

_____

_____

_____

_____

_____

Learn the lesson so that you maybe released from the trial.

SIX-STEP PROCESS

Take your time with these steps. Be patient with yourself and enjoy the process. Remember gratitude is the key!

BE SURE TO SLOW DOWN

Allow time for thinking. Sometimes when we're too busy we stop the possibilities of our breakthrough. Proper timing and proper pacing is essential.

KEEP PUSHING

When you think you've gone as far as you can, keep going & push yourself. A breakthrough in life happens as you knock down and pass your barriers.

TAKE YOUR MIND ON AN ADVENTURE

Now is the time to become a child again. Deliberately step outside of your comfort zone. You are the change you are seeking in life.

EXPAND YOUR THINKING BY LISTENING TO OTHERS

Listen to those who are where you want to be. Listen to those who have gone through many breakthroughs in life and are succeeding.

PROPER PLANNING

Some people strategize their way through their breakthrough. You have to find strategies that fit you. Your strategy is your unique plan and your method to reach your goal.

MAKE YOUR STORY COUNT

Everyone has a story to tell! Make yours count! Whether you believe it does or not, someone needs to hear your story.

TAKE ACTION NOW

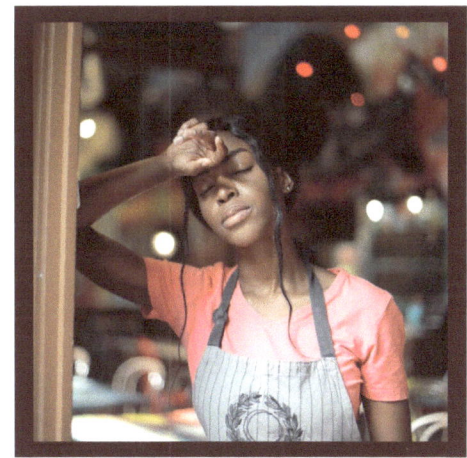

SLOW DOWN AND GIVE YOURSELF SPACE

Take a moment to clear your schedule and rest your mind. Make you a priority! You deserve the freedom.

A CALL TO ACTION

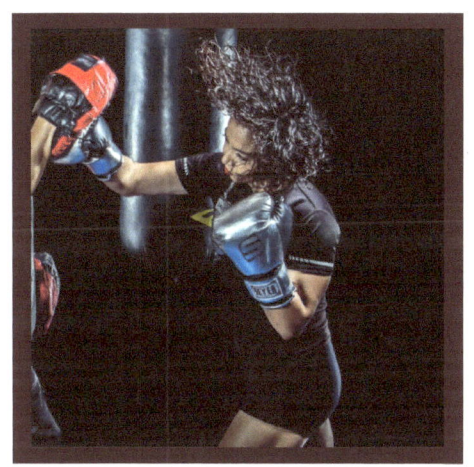

KEEP PUSHING

Witness your inner greatness. You are the best. You have what it takes to get to the finish line. You MUST believe in yourself! Nothing and no one can stop you, but yourself.

A CALL TO ACTION

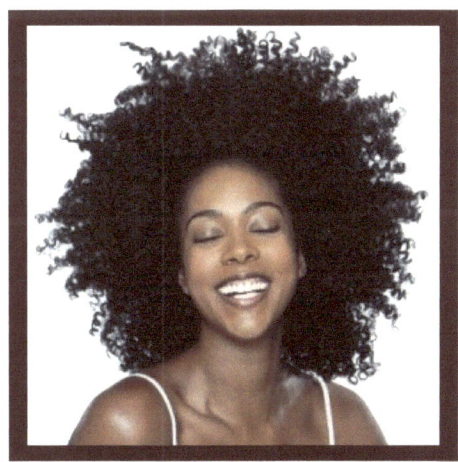

YOU WILL WIN!

Declare your win! Say aloud, "I WILL WIN! I WILL CLEAR MY MIND AND MY SPACE. I WILL FIGHT TO CROSS THE FINISH LINE!"

A CALL TO ACTION

Take Your Mind On An Adventure

When we were children we often imagined ourselves doing the unimaginable. We took giant leaps and bound forward. Place your mind where you want your reality to be. Use the following page to write about your adventure and keep reflecting back on it.

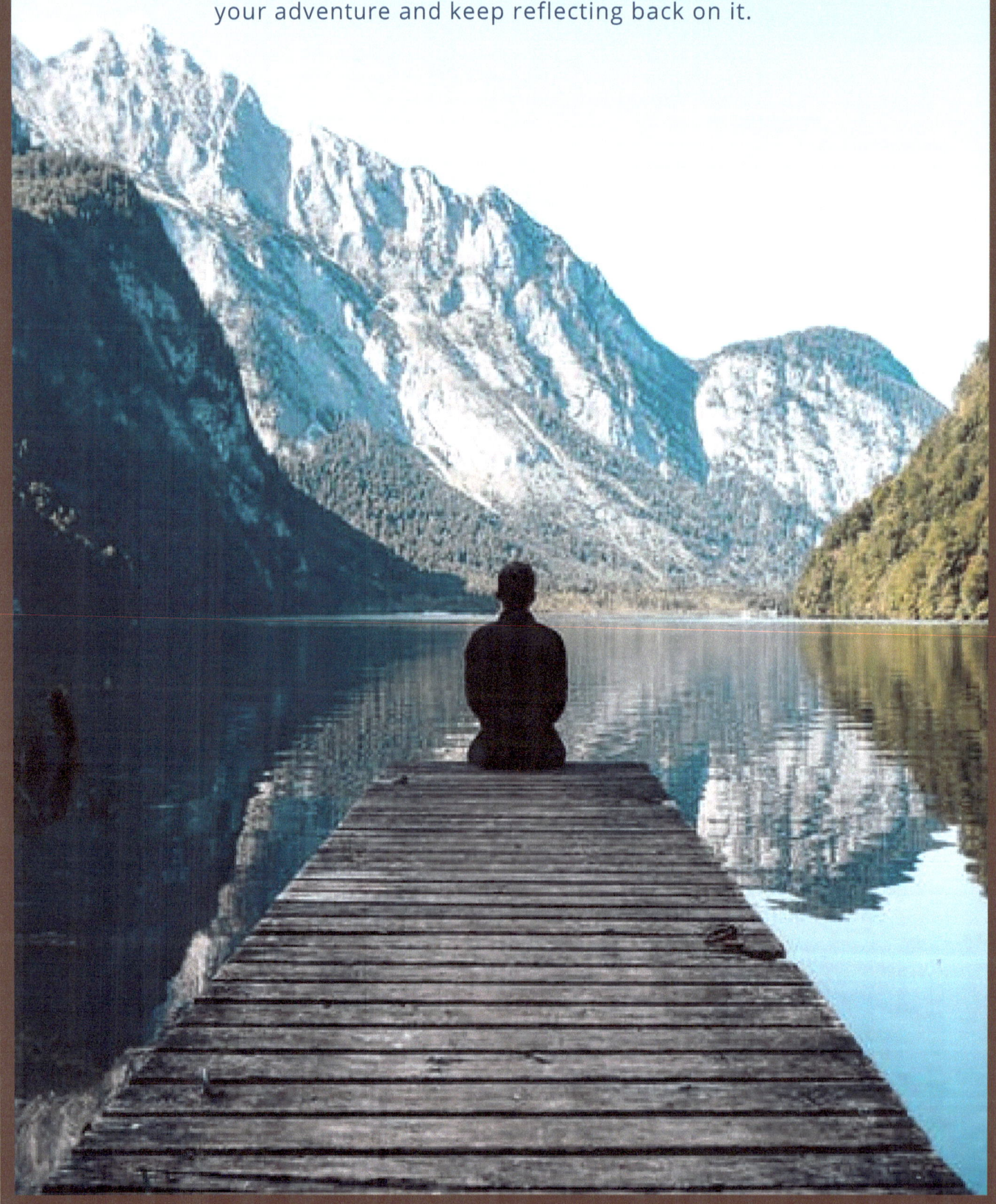

MY ADVENTURE

EXPAND YOUR THINKING

Studying other's and their accomplishments can be done through personal conversations, watching videos, reading books, listening to audio books, etc. It is an encouraging experience when you see others accomplishing what you are trying to accomplish.

Pick up from their experiences what is useful to you. Wise people study others. They understand this journey of life is not to be done alone. It's all about who and what will help you on your journey.

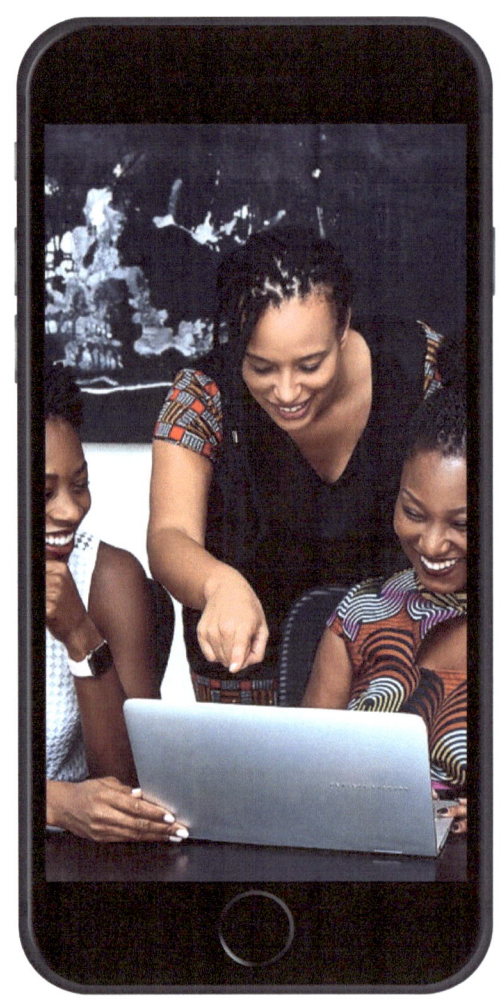

WHAT ARE THE PROS OF YOUR JOURNEY?

WHAT ARE THE CONS OF YOUR JOURNEY?

WHO'S FEEDING YOUR MIND?

GOD

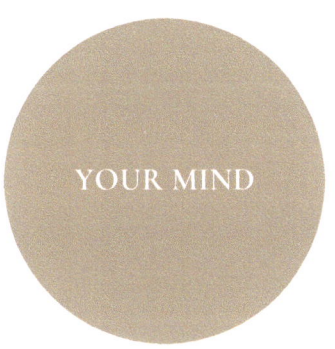

NOTES

PROPER PLANNING-
RESEARCH TIME

WHAT IS YOUR STRATEGY TO GET YOU THROUGH YOUR BREAKTHROUGH?
WHAT WORKS BEST FOR YOU?

_____

_____

STEPS

WHAT IS YOUR PLAN B STRATEGY?

_____

_____

STEPS

MAKE YOUR STORY COUNT

You may think you have a past filled with negative experiences. Guess what? You are not alone. Your breakthrough is a rescue misson for yourself and someone else. Write some bullet points of your life's story.

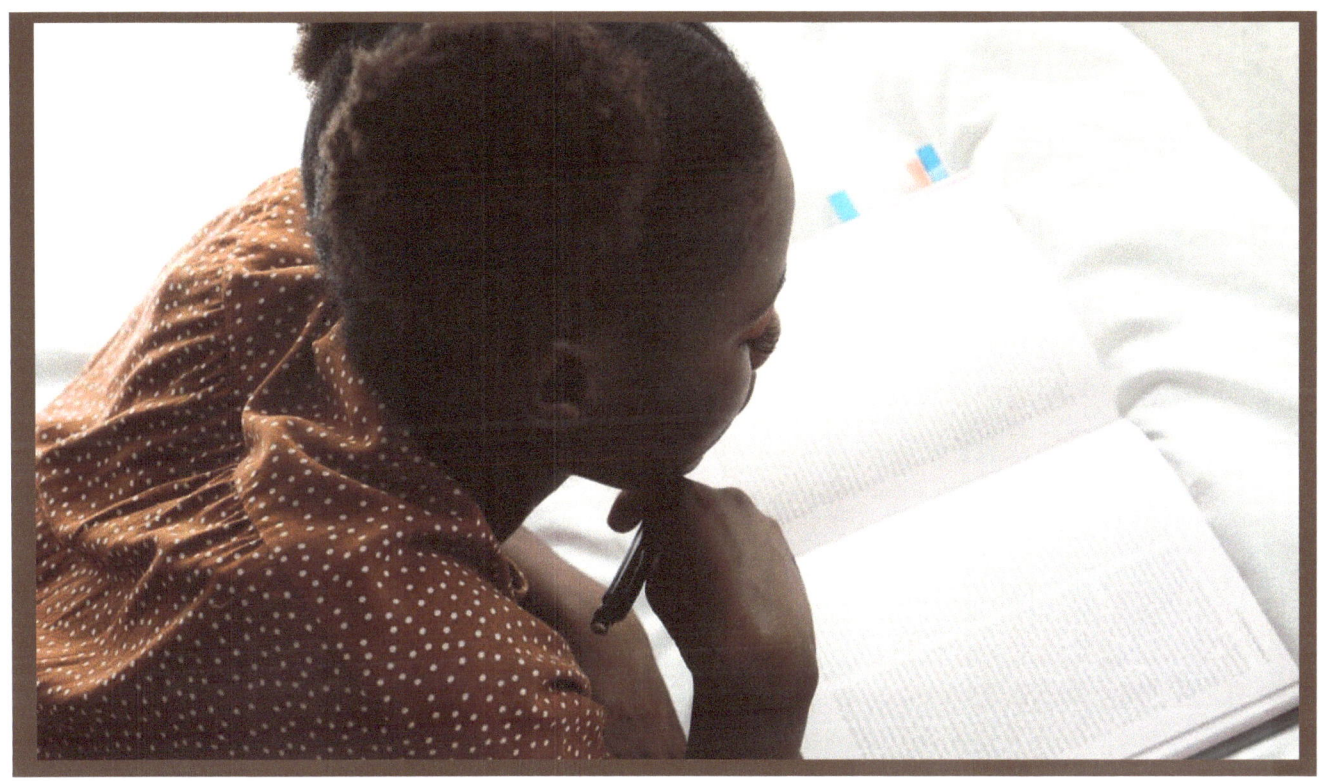

POSITIVE EXPERIENCES   NEGATIVE EXPERIENCES

MY
SUCCESS STORY

Write a summary of your success story and place your picture in the circle.

SELF-CARE!

I have learned throughout the years of my life, that if you do not take care of yourself, you are not fully capable of taking care of others and you are creating a recipe for self-destruction. We must be true to ourselves. We must fall in love with the beautiful vessel God created us to be. Once you identify who you are, you will see that you are a unique creation of God. There is no other like you.

Stop comparing yourself to others. Take this module and use it to help you fall deeper in love with yourself. You will create your own recipe's for self-care and you will have access to some you may find beneficial. The goal is to learn how to take better care of yourself and to love the unique essence God created you to be.

You will not settle. You will develop your best self. This process takes time and may not be easy. You can do it. Take it from a person who has been through these steps. It was a challenge, but I welcomed it and enjoyed the process!

THREE-STEP PROCESS

Before beginning any module, you must complete the three step process. This process is to help you enter into the state of being for healing.

STEP ONE...

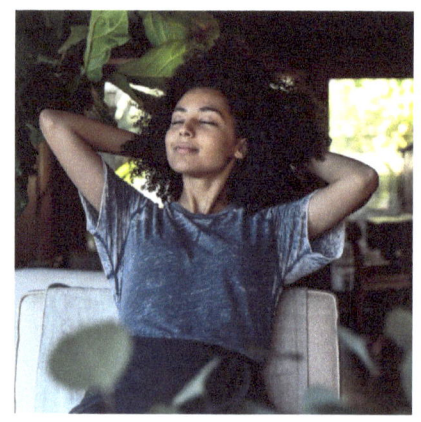

Settle into a comfortable place and breathe mindfully. Rest for two to three minutes. You should begin to feel relaxed.

STEP TWO...

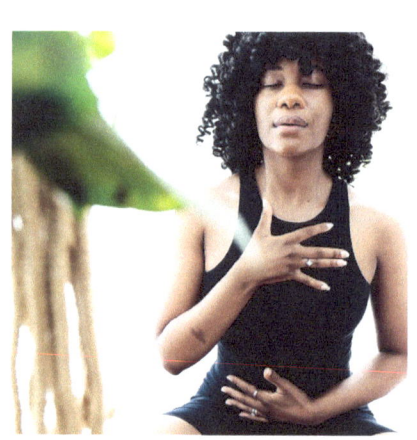

Pick an area of your body to focus on for another two to three minutes. (forehead, toes, lips, hands, etc.) Keep controlling your breathing.

STEP THREE...

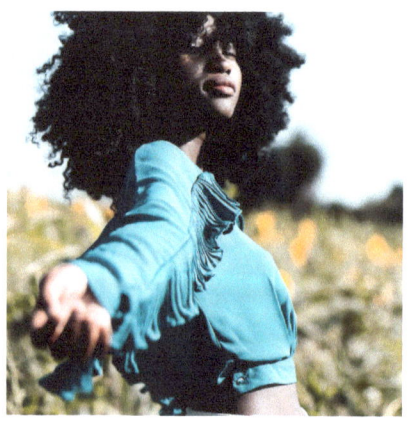

Say to yourself,
I am ready to heal.
I am ready to grow.
I am ready to become my best self!

YOUR EMPOWERMENT

WOMEN IN HISTORY

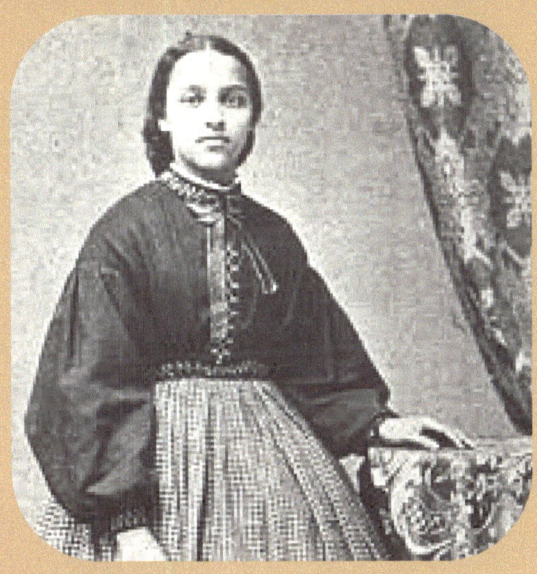

I was the first black woman to gradute from an established American college. I was the first Black Principal at Dunbar High School.
I AM MARY JANE PATTERSON!

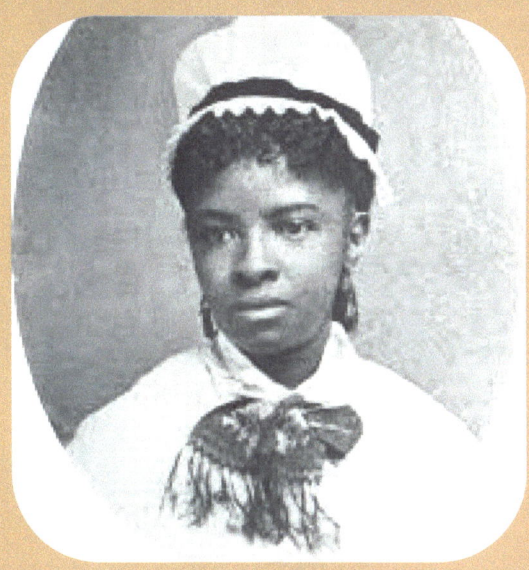

I am the first black nurse. I became one of the first black women to register to vote in Boston. I was the founding member of the American Nurses Association.
I AM MARY ELIZA MAHONEY!

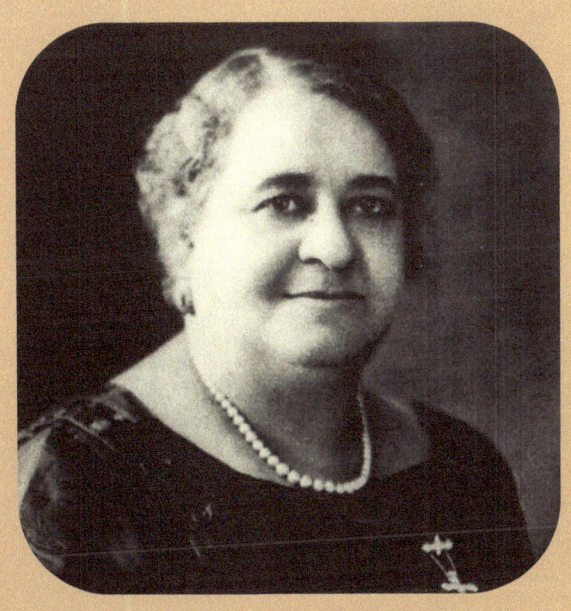

I was the daugther of a former slave. I attended public school in Richmond, VA. I broke race and gender barriers. I became the first Black person and the first female to establish and serve as president of a United States bank.
I AM MAGGIE LENA WALKER!

NOW IS THE TIME TO LOVE ON YOU!

We are jewels of God's treasure chest. Some of us may be dull. Some of us may even be broken. But it is through His Word that we are polished and mended. We are the best! We onluy need to strengthen our relationship with The One Who is the key to our success. He is The Light in our darkness, The Water that quenches our thirst. He is The Food that nourishes our existence. The Oxygen that feeds our cells. He is our beginning and through Him we will have no end.

With this module you will create your loving, healing space with you and God. Enjoy every moment!

THESE ACTIVITIES MAKE ME FEEL FREE:

_____

_____

_____

_____

_____

I illuminate the world!
I shine!
I am God's light!

PRAYER IS A GIFT FROM GOD

Prayer heals. It strengthens, it builds our faith, our courage, develops our intimate relationship with God, and provides peace. Just having God on your mind is a prayer. Take in His breath and feed off of His word. Heal your soul.

WHAT WORDS WILL HEAL YOUR SOUL?

_____

_____

PERSONAL PRAYER

LOVE ON ME POSTER BOARD

In the beginning was The Word. Create a poster board filled with messages that empower, inspire and foster love of self. NO IMAGES ONLY WORDS. You can refer to page 125 of "The Power to Break Generational Pain" for additional guidance on this activity.

FEED YOUR SOUL

START Believe
adventure
Love COURAGE
Focus DREAM
FINISH
Laughter play
EXPLORE
Enjoy CREATE
wander Strength

FOUR STEPS TO REST

Write down four necessary steps that you will do to clear your mind.

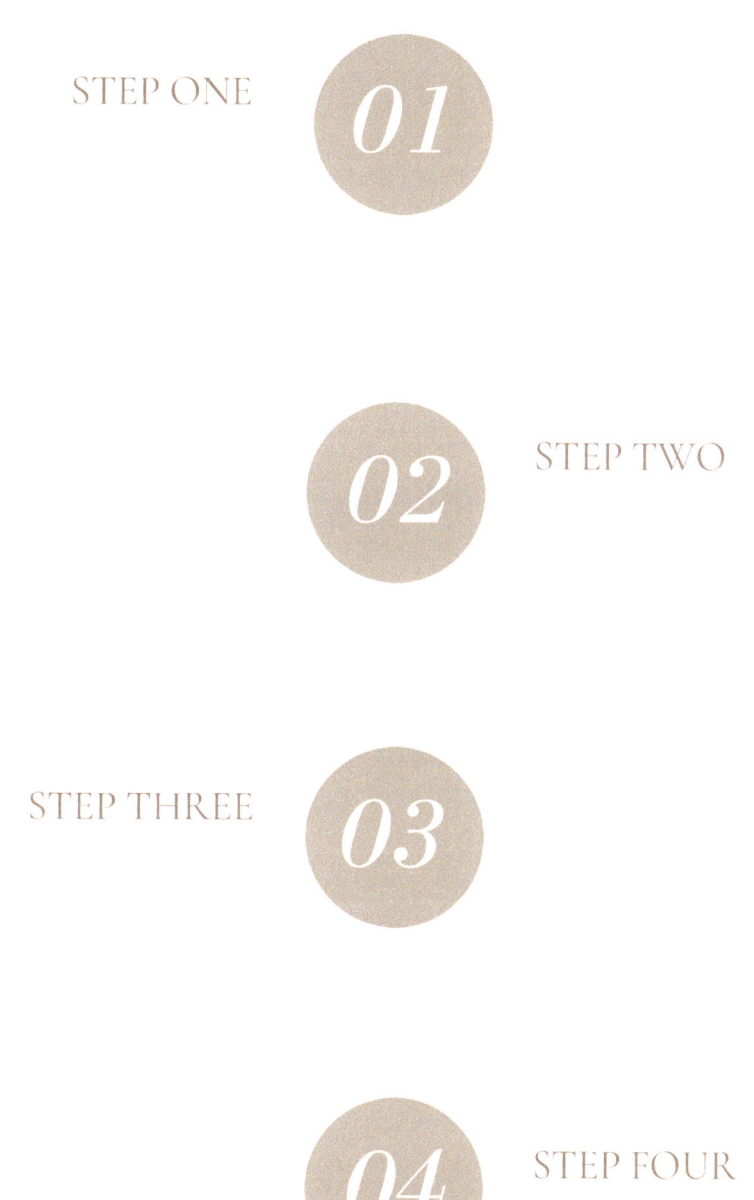

STEP ONE
01

02
STEP TWO

STEP THREE
03

04
STEP FOUR

Organization Challenge

Challenge yourself to organize and prioritze your daily schedule. Write down your a list of your tasks everyday.

Reading Challenge

Challenge yourself to read books that feed your mind for growth and development. Choose books in areas you desire to grow.

New & Old Challenge

Challenge yourself to form new healthy habits and to get rid of the old ones. Tell yourself bad habits don't exist in your life anymore.

Eat To Live Challenge

Challenge yourself to eat a good diet. Stop feeding your body junk. You will no longer engage in behavior that is self-destructive.

COPING WITH STRESS

When we're under stress, our perspective narrows and our bodies begin to shut down. Do these activities to deal with stress.

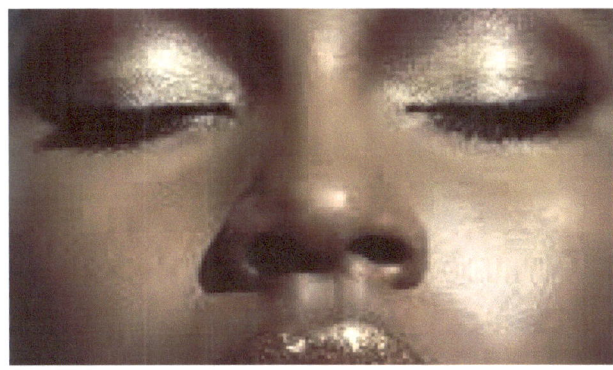

CALM YOUR MIND

Breathe, listen to running water, take a warm bath, listen to soothing music, get in touch with nature.

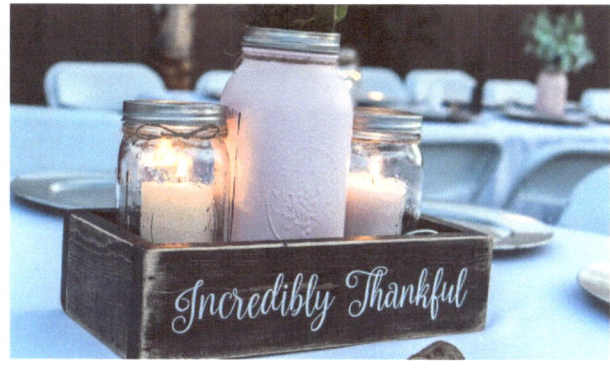

SPIRITUAL

Meditate, study God's Word, list five things you are grateful for, journal, spend time with nature, pray.

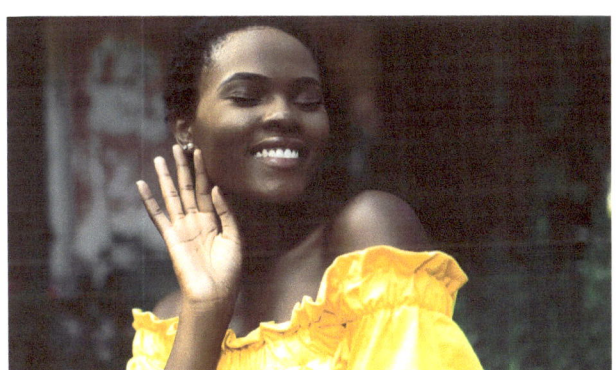

EMOTIONS

Confront your feelings. Cry, laugh, practice self-compassion. Control the pattern of your thoughts.

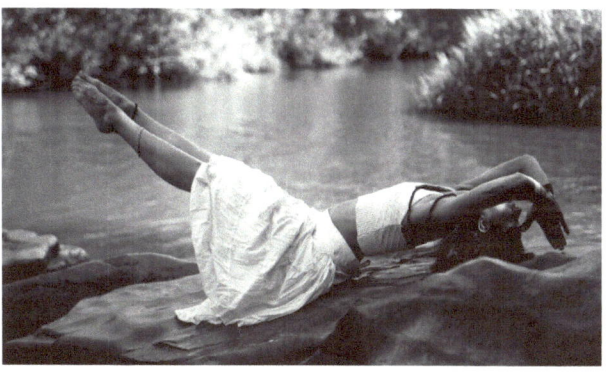

PHYSICAL

Practice yoga, dance, sing, stretch, go for a walk, take a nap with a clear mind. Create a basic workout plan.

MY FAVORITE LIST FOR SELF CARE

BALANCED BREATHING

I do focused breathing for ten minutes a day. I sit comfortably with proper posture and breathe in for a count of seven and breathe out for a count of seven.

WALKING THROUGH NATURE

I walk through a garden filled with trees or walk by a body of water enjoying the scenery of nature.

EXPRESSING GRATITUDE

I thank God for His creations. I thank God for life. I thank God for pain, joy, laughter, growth and His inspiration. I thank God for His mercy and His love. I practice keeping God on my mind.

RELAXING

I take a day and do absolutely nothing except love on me. I may just sit still and allow my body to rest. may give yourself a pedicure, read God's Word or a good book.

WATCHING MOVIES

I cuddle up and watch my favorite movies or TV Shows all day. I eat my favorite comfort food (in moderation).

YOUR FAVORITE LIST FOR SELF CARE

01

02

03

04

05

NOTES

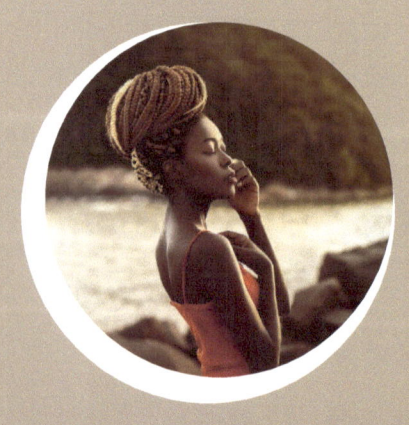

No matter what type of trial you may be experiencing, don't let go of the only one who has the power to see you through it. Become one with your creator.

ENDING ASSESSMENT

Take this assessment to see the progress you have made after completing this workbook.

	YES	NO
Do you feel you can properly handle fear, anxiety or panic?		
Do you now have a better way to handle pain inflicted on you?		
Can you now prevent yourself from becoming overwhelmed by your circumstances?		
Do you now experience restful nights?		
Do you feel you have the tools to rid your life of doubt and depression?		
Do you believe you are healing?		

YOUR CHECKLIST

Create a checklist to help you stay focused on what you need to continue your healing.

YOUR CHECKLIST ITEM

NOTES

YOUR CHECKLIST ITEM

YOUR CHECKLIST ITEM

YOUR CHECKLIST ITEM

YOUR CHECKLIST ITEM

YOUR PERSONAL
TESTIMONY

RESOURCE LIBRARY

WHY I AM ENOUGH

Your daily inspiration! This book is fillied with inspiration and healing. Some of the quotes in this workbook came from "Why I Am Enough".

ORDER YOUR COPY
WWW.HEAL-THYLIFE.COM

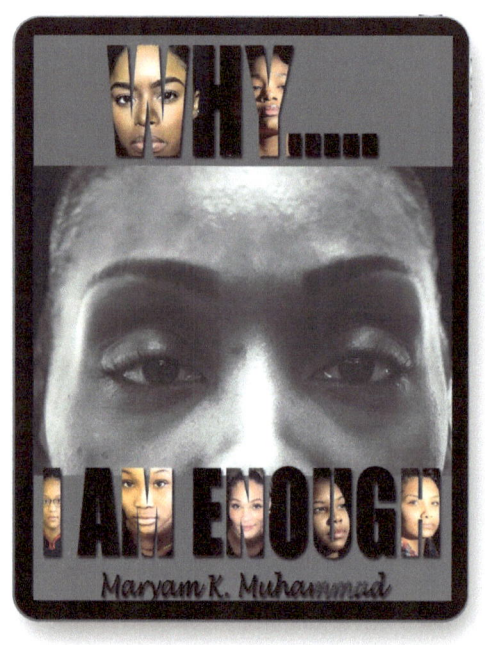

LADIES... LET'S TALK NUTRITION

This workbook is designed to help you become aware of what's happening in your body so that you may make healthier choices. It is all about you! There are colorful and easy to follow recipes, information on diseases, mental wellness steps and more.

ORDER YOUR COPY
WWW.HEAL-THYLIFE.COM

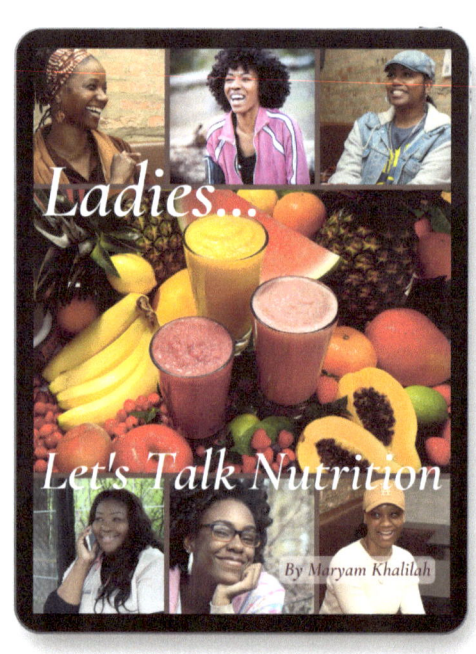

CREATE YOUR OWN
RESOURCE LIBRARY

YOUR RESOURCE NAME

YOUR RESOURCE NAME

YOUR RESOURCE NAME

YOUR RESOURCE NAME

THANK YOU!

I thank God for blessing me with the mind and guidance to create this workbook for you. I am not the healer, God is! I thank you for being courageous enough to take the steps to heal your life. Always keep God in mind. Remember, when your inner self awakens and removes insecurities and you strengthen your self-love, you are on your way to becoming completely healed.

You were born on purpose with a purpose. God has a plan for you. Walk with Him. His essence is in you. Pull on it and use it. Only settle on God's energy from this day forward!

Claim your victory. You're already winning!

Maryam Khalilah

xoxo

STAY IN TOUCH

INSTAGRAM @HTLC19	TWITTER @HTLC19
WWW.HEAL-THYLIFE.COM	FACEBOOK @HTLC19